DIET OVER 50

---

2 books in 1:

Intermittent Fasting Over 50 + Keto for woman over 50.

160 recipes, and 30-Day Weight Loss Plans for Beginners, Complete With a 30-Day Meal Plan and Physical Exercises to Maintain Ketosis

---

SHANA KATHY

Table of Contents

INTRODUCTION 7

CHAPTER 1 THE MAGICAL DIET OF INTERMITTENT FASTING 50: WHY TO TRY IT 11

CHAPTER 2 BENEFITS OF INTERMITTENT FASTING 19

CHAPTER 3 MEAL PLAN FOR 14 DAYS 29

CHAPTER 4 INTERMITTENT FASTING AND SUPPLEMENTS 31

CHAPTER 5 OTHER TIPS TO FOLLOW TO MAKE IF MORE EFFECTIVE 35

CHAPTER 6. THE INTERMITTENT FASTING TYPE 45

CHAPTER 7 HOW TO PLAN 53

CHAPTER 8 DIET IN MENOPAUSE 57

CHAPTER 9. MYTHS ABOUT INTERMITTENT FASTING 67

CHAPTER 10 COMMON MISTAKES 73

CHAPTER 11 INTERMITTENT FASTING AND EXERCISE 83

CHAPTER 12 SPIRULINA ALGAE: THE SUPPLEMENT THAT HELPS YOUR FAST 89

CHAPTER 13. WHAT TO AVOID AND WHAT TO EAT 93

CHAPTER 14 BREAKFAST RECIPES 101

CHAPTER 15. LUNCH RECIPES 131

CHAPTER 16. SNACK RECIPES 159

CONCLUSION 185

INTRODUCTION 190

CHAPTER 1: WHAT YOU NEED TO KNOW ABOUT THE KETOGENIC DIET 192

CHAPTER 2: BASIC ITEMS THAT SHOULD BE IN YOUR PANTRY (OR ON YOUR SHOPPING LIST) **202**

CHAPTER 3: KETO RECIPES FOR BREAKFAST 206

CHAPTER 4: RECIPES FOR LUNCH 276

CHAPTER 5: KETO DINNER RECIPES 344

CHAPTER 6: KETO SNACKS 406

CHAPTER 7: 30-DAY MEAL PREP FOR BEGINNERS AND 7-DAY EXERCISE PLAN 466

BOOK 1
INTERMITTENT FASTING FOR WOMEN OVER 50

The Winning Formula to Lose Weight, Unlock Metabolism and Delay Aging. It Only Takes a Few Hours without Food to Obtain Immediate Results

SHANA KATHY

Introduction

Fasting is an ancient practice that has been practiced by many cultures and religions, such as Islam's month-long Ramadan or the Jewish Yom Kippur. In a nutshell, intermittent fasting means not ingesting any calories for extended periods of time. While most people think of this as abstaining from all food and liquid, it can also consist of restricting calorie intake on certain days, which is called intermittent fasting.

IF has been found to have many benefits for both men and women, such as improved weight loss, better blood sugar control, increased focus, improved skin complexion, weight maintenance, reduced anxiety, depression and blood pressure. It is particularly effective for older adults as it helps improve insulin sensitivity, which promotes a healthy metabolism and helps the body better utilize blood sugar.

Intermittent fasting is also great for hormonal health. By helping optimize insulin sensitivity and blood sugar levels, your hormones are able to run more efficiently. This includes helpful hormones like leptin that help manage your appetite and ghrelin that stimulates your body's hunger response. These hormones are critical in managing weight by getting you into a healthy calorie-burning balance.

Women and Intermittent Fasting

There are different types of intermittent fasting, yet it is most effective if done on a daily basis. One of the ways that women can do this is to have a fast day and eat according to their body's needs. Does this sound like you? A fast day means you have one day where you don't eat any food or drink anything but water. You might consider fasting every other day, alternating with non-fast days, where you eat as much as feels good for your body.

How long should these fasting days be? It can vary based on how clean your diet has been and how many calories that meal the previous day has. Ideally, it will be from 10 to 14 hours. The general recommendation is not to go over 16 hours.

As you can imagine, women who are older may find fasting difficult and should consult their health care practitioner before trying any form of fasting. Women who are pregnant or breastfeeding should also consult their physician prior to trying a fast day.

Remember, this is not an extreme form of fasting. The goal is to simply help you realize how you feel when you are not eating or drinking anything. You may be surprised at the benefits that can come from a 10- 12-hour fast day.

This type of intermittent fasting will also show you how much food is truly necessary for sustaining yourself on a daily basis.

You can then work to incorporate and minimize your food intake while still eating the foods you enjoy. Keep in mind, however, that the results of fasting do not come from skipping a meal or eating less. They come from changing to a healthier lifestyle that includes healthier foods and portion sizes.

Another great way to get some of the benefits of fasting is to simply restrict your calorie intake on a given day. This can be done by restricting your daily calorie intake by 20 percent. While this is more than what most experts recommend, if you are already eating well and working out regularly, it may be the perfect kick-start to your weight loss journey.

The first fast day in this protocol is generally done one to two weeks after the beginning of your weight loss journey. This way, if you are already on a meal plan, you will soon be able to begin incorporating fasting into your lifestyle. If you are not on a meal plan, I would recommend consulting with your health care professional before starting the intermittent fasting protocol.

Chapter 1
The Magical Diet of Intermittent Fasting 50: Why to Try It

Improved Cognitive Function and Clarity

Fasting has great beneficial consequences for balanced cognitive processes. The most well-known benefit is in cellular activation of autophagy, which is a cell cleansing process. Note that fasting has anti-seizure effects.

Improvement in Hormone Profile

Many people avoid intermittent fasting due to the assumption that it would lead to deterioration of health. This isn't always the case for those who do take part in intermittent fasting. Studies have shown that fasting does not negatively impact those who conduct daily physical activities, particularly if you cut down on your carbs you fast and are in a ketosis state. Studies have shown that performing high-intensity exercise on fasted days can lead to higher metabolic adaptations.

Reduces Inflammation

Intermittent fasting (IF) encourages autophagy due to the body's self-maintenance method. Killing off old cells is objectionable because it's hard to do. However, it can be used as an alternative to other methods of eliminating unwanted dirt from the human body. It's a normal way the human body cleans and restores itself. Damaged or old cells may lead to inflammation. Intermittent fasting can be an efficient way to minimize inflammation in the body.

Supports Healthy Bodily Functions

Intermittent fasting is a time-saving way of eating that allows time to digest and get other things done. When you eat food, your body is given time to consume and use it for energy. In modern society, people often overeat and are negatively influenced by issues of lifestyle, which have contributed to constant eating. So, our systems can get overloaded and we can't process anything we want to. This can lead to you not getting enough nutrition, storing fats, and struggling to produce healthy levels of natural hormones and chemicals within your body.

Polycystic Ovarian Syndrome and Intermittent Fasting

Getting polycystic ovaries is fairly common in women. The disease can trigger a hormone imbalance, which can affect women adversely. Many women experience weight gain from AIDS and weight gain from other diseases. While there are not too many reports on the impact of intermittent fasting on the metabolic disorder, there is evidence that the combination of intermittent fasting and a low-carbohydrate ketogenic diet resulted in weight loss for polycystic ovarian syndrome patients. There is potential hope that intermittent fasting can be used to mitigate the impact of hormonal and metabolic disorders. Time and further study will decide whether or not intermittent fasting has a role to play in treating this disease.

Change in Cell Function

While fasting, various biochemical and physiological changes take place in your body. After exercise, your body will begin the process of cellular repair, and hormone levels will shift. Lower levels of Uric Acid give the body greater access to stored fat. You will note a decrease in the amount of insulin because it makes it easier to metabolize fat and burn it, thus decreasing weight. An increase in the human growth hormone helps to increase lean muscle and burn more fat than usual. Damaged cells are processed, and other processes of cellular repair kick in. Also, several changes take place within the genes and molecules that protect you against disease.

Improved Sleep

There is at least one experimental study that has shown that people who become used to intermittent fasting have improved sleep quality. The explanation of why this happens is possibly complicated, but there have been conclusive demonstrations that intermittent fasting over an extended period assists in good sleep.

Mood and Motivation

The study of the effect of intermittent fasting on mood and motivation is in its infancy. There is a lack of research on large populations using the statistical techniques of randomized controls. However, some studies have demonstrated that intermittent fasting does improve both mood and motivation in a surprisingly short period. As there is profound controversy about the pharmacological treatments of people's mental state, any treatment which has no side effects and many potential benefits must be considered seriously.

Cardiovascular Health

Intermittent fasting leads to a reduction in weight. For this and other reasons, it leads to an improvement in cardiovascular health. The cause of such disease is usually atherosclerosis, the deposit of plaque in blood vessel walls. The dysfunction of the endothelium, which is a thin lining of the blood vessels, causes atherosclerosis. A healthy endothelium works to prevent this insidious deposit.

The endothelium is not doing its job properly if plaque builds up. Obesity, especially where the fat deposits are in the abdominal area, leads in many cases to this buildup of plaque.

Other causes of this deposit are stress and inflammation. Intermittent fasting assists in the reduction of these, as well as obesity. Some studies show improvements in all risk factors for cardiovascular health.

Gut Health

Scientists are increasingly aware of the essential role of microorganisms in the human digestive system. These are known as the microbiome. There are trillions of them, and they are in other parts of the body, apart from the gut. Many diseases originate in the gut, not only illnesses concerning that part of the body but also of the brain, the heart, and all other regions of the body.

There is research on mice that caloric restriction improves that part of the microbiome in the gut. The effect of this is to prolong the life of the mice. In humans, the effects of dietary changes are very swift, even as short as hours. Studies are currently being done to verify that the real effects of intermittent fasting observed in the gut health of mice are true for humans as well.

Weight Loss

The key advantage of this diet is weight loss. When you follow intermittent fasting, the number of meals you eat will be reduced. When you eat less, the calories you consume will decrease as well. When a person's insulin levels decrease, growth hormone and norepinephrine levels increase. These two hormones facilitate the breakdown of stored fat. The body burns more calories from food when you fast, and this helps you stay in shape. The effect of intermittent fasting is twofold: By increasing your metabolic rate, it helps your body to burn fat and increase productivity. Reducing how much you consume food will help you lose weight.

Lowers the Risk of Diabetes

The most common health problem that plagues humanity these days, apart from obesity, is diabetes. High blood sugar leads to insulin resistance in the body. Intermittent fasting helps to reduce blood sugar and therefore helps reduce insulin resistance in the body. When a person's body becomes immune to insulin, they typically experience elevated blood sugar levels, and the cycle of hyperglycemia follows. If you opt for this diet, you can successfully reverse this condition.

It Boosts Your Metabolic Rate

Studies show that staying in a fasted state leads to a spike in the hormone norepinephrine. This hormone increases your basal metabolic rate and burns fat. On top of that, once you enter your eating window, your metabolism still stays at an elevated level. You are essentially burning excess fat even when eating!

Convert Your Body Fat

Many people are unaware that they have two distinct forms of fat. This fat isn't all the same. There is safe and unhealthy body fat of various amounts in different individuals. White fat, which builds up with an over intake of excess calories, is harmful to health, contributes to aging, and ultimately leads to disease.

On the one hand, brown body fat protects the body from injury while at the same time preserving health. By following intermittent fasting, you not only lose weight through weight loss but also detoxifies the toxic white fat into healthy brown fat. Additionally, brown fat burns away excess white fat, which stops you from producing white fat, and maintains a healthy weight.

Improve Muscle Health

Many people get excited about the temporary weight reduction they experience when trying the crash diet. That is until they stop losing weight and eventually give up on a diet. But, most of the weight loss people achieve on these diets is not fat loss but water weight and muscle weight. Since muscle weighs more than fat tissue, even a small amount of muscle or fat loss can make a significant difference on the scale.

As crash diets promote malnutrition, it naturally leads to muscle loss, which negatively affects your health and strength as you age. After all, your muscles are in much more than your arms. They are surrounding your entire body, and even your heart is a muscle! As you lose muscle, your health and energy will be dramatically affected, and it is essential to regain this as you age if you want to improve your health. Thankfully, studies have found that when compared to dieting, intermittent fasting not only leads to more weight loss than dieting, but it also causes much less muscle loss. This means your muscles will become much healthier, especially if you actively work out while you practice fasting.

Boosted Energy

The mitochondria, which are within our mitochondrial cells, are the powerhouse of the cell. It is the mitochondria that allow us to use a variety of fuel sources from the food we eat as fuel, as well as ketones. While other cells in the body may only be able to utilize one or two fuel types for energy, the mitochondrial is incredibly versatile to be able to use all kinds of fuel. When one fasts for prolonged periods of time (or is on a low-carb/ketogenic diet), a person's body starts to produce ketones. These are then used to cross the blood-brain barrier and power the brain, even when glucose is not accessible. When you are in this fasted state of ketosis, the body will also increase the number of mitochondrial cells within your body, replacing non-mitochondrial cells with mitochondrial cells, allowing for more of your cells to be fueled by any fuel source.

Since the mitochondrial fuel ninety percent of the human body, by increasing the number of these cells, you can naturally increase your energy. Not only will your physical energy increase, but your mental functioning and energy will, as well. This is great news for many people who lose energy as they age.

Chapter 2
Benefits of Intermittent Fasting

Good Health Enhancement

All over the past, various societies had discovered the advantageous effects on health and general welfare of reducing food consumption for definite periods, either for religious motives or when food was rare. The first extensive systematic study, published by Mc Cay et al. in 1935, highlighted the restricted eating diets and their capability to expand lifespan. Mc Cay explained that feeding rats with a diet comprising of edible cellulose dramatically expand both the mean and maximum life-span in these animals. Many studies have verified this consequence and extended it to mice and other species like fruit flies, nematodes, water fleas, spiders, and fish. So dietary changes affect life-span and health-span, then the time of our lives. We have a disorder/pathology-free disposition.

We will likewise analyze through which molecular mechanisms the points of interest, all in all, living beings, of dietary utilization changes are determined. Modification of this main dietary routine, now known as a caloric limitation, is the most effective way of expanding the lifespan of mammals without genetically changing them. In particular, intermittent fasting has also been explained to extend lifespan and have beneficial health effects.

Rodents upheld on calorie-limited diets are usually lesser and leaner. They have less body fat, and smaller major organs than ad libitum fed animals. They are probably more active, which may bring about the need to search for food. The typical age-concerned reduction in physical activity decreases in the calorie-limited animal. However, these animals are more susceptible to cold temperatures that affect death in small mammals.

Crucially, both caloric limitation and intermittent fasting can reduce the severity of critical factors for diseases such as diabetes and cardiovascular disease in rodents. In many studies, the occasional fasting routine application ends in an approximately 20 to 30% reduction in caloric consumption over time. Preservation of rats on this alternate day CL feeding routine for 2 to 4 months enhances hippocampal neurons' resistance to chemically produced degeneration. This progressive impairment of hippocampal neurons is also related to hitting learning and memory preservation in a water maze spatial learning task. Thus, these dietary routines could have an essential benefit for incapacitating and prevalent neurodegenerative disorders such as Alzheimer's, Huntington's, and Parkinson's diseases.

Intermittent Fasting Effect on Lipid Metabolism

Survival and maintenance of species steadiness amongst others depend on their accessibility to food. That is why living organisms have progressed with many adaptive procedures that permit them to live periods of starvation. Some microorganisms or animals in the periods where they do not have access to food are dormant; for example, yeasts stay in a stationary phase, while mammals use the liver and adipose tissue for sustenance. These set up an energy storeroom for them that permits them to live in periods of deprivation. Fats production is an essential mechanism of the human body. The fats' amount varied due to the body's conditions, and their role satisfied the organism's request. One of the essential functions is that of the stoppage and energy function.

The adipocytes preserve energy. Under specific circumstances, they are discharged from them under the effect of the enzyme lipase. After the consumption of a meal, the amount of glucose in the body enhances. Then within a few hours, it reverts to the condition it was before dinner. The number of ketones is less because the glycogen stored in the liver not reduce. Throughout the intermittent fasting diet, which consists of informing fasting periods, there are noticeable metabolic variations in the body. During the day, all food consumed in 6 to 8 hours increases the glucose level in about 6 hours after a meal but remains low for the remaining 16 hours until the next day. During the 6 to 8 hours in an eighteen-fasting gap, ketones increase. The human body adjusts to such periods of fasting. In the instant of hunger, adaptation procedures start to gain energy. In a fasting gap, when glucose consumes, the body begins to use ketones that elevate due to fatty acid alterations. Fatty acids and ketones develop the necessary resource of energy for cells. This changeover is called intermittent metabolic switching (IMS) or glucose-ketone (G-to-K) switchover. While the body is desisting from food, the amount of glucose, which is the primary energy substrate, reduces. Then it is consumed the glycogen stocks in the liver, stimulating the reaction of gluconeogenesis.

Moreover, insulin and IGF-1 (insulin-like growth factor-1) levels decrease in the blood, and glucagon levels elevate. The lipolysis of the fatty acids produces triacylglycerol and diacylglycerol. They moved to the liver cells, where they changed into β-hydroxybutyrate (BHB) and acetoacetate (AcAc) in the β-oxidation reaction and are further freed into the blood and consumed as a source of energy for body cells, involving the brain. Such biochemical alteration goes with cellular and molecular adaptations of neuronal nets in the brain. The consequence is the development of their functionality and resistance to stress, injuries, and diseases. The above biochemical alterations of lipids and following the intermittent fasting result in weight reduction and lipid parameters variations. According to studies showed by Surabhi Bhutani et al., during the usage of alternative days on an unfilled stomach, the alternate-day fasting for 2 to 3 weeks presented a decrease in body weight by 3%. Prolonged application of alternate-day fasting indicated a reduction of 8% and decreased fat mass in the viscera. Besides, the levels of total cholesterol triglycerides and low-density cholesterol (LDL) and these molecules' size decrease the alterations in these factors reduce the risk of growing coronary heart disease.

The Influence of Intermittent Fasting on Inflammatory Biomarkers

Atherosclerosis is a significant danger of pathogenicity and death in both developed and developing countries. It is a chronic inflammatory disease in which atherosclerotic plaque forms in arterial vessels, which causes sclerosis of the walls and tightening of the arteries. One of the principal dangerous factors regards the high levels of low-density lipoproteins LDL. These levels stimulate an inflammatory response and adhesion to the endothelium of blood leukocytes, basically monocytes. They roam to the inner membrane of the vessels and change into macrophages. Stimulated cells discharge factors that add to smooth muscle cell migration from the medial to the inner. Vascular smooth muscle cells reproduce and release extracellular matrix proteins. This pathology's clinical symptoms are ischemic heart disease, peripheral artery disease, and ischemic stroke. It is accountable for severe myocardial infarction and cerebrovascular events. It is also responsible for most deaths resulting from cardiovascular causes in the world.

There is a further gathering of lipids both within cells and extracellularly. The majority of critical factors for cardiovascular diseases and aspects of atherosclerosis may be reduced, also by intermittent fasting. Inflammation is an essential element of development. Inflammatory factors, such as homocysteine, interleukin 6 (IL6), take part in atherosclerotic plaque development. The research conducted by Aksungar et al. verified the fasting influence on decreasing the amount of the above-stated proinflammatory factors.

Forty healthy volunteers joined the trial with the right body mass index (BMI), who fasted in Ramadan, and 28 with BMI index, which did not fast. Venous blood tested to analyze the concentration of the above-described proinflammatory factors were gathered one week earlier the start of Ramadan, in the last week of fasting, and three weeks after.

Adiponectin is a collagen-like plasma protein whose concentration reduces in the course of atherosclerosis, insulin resistance, diabetes, and coronary disease. The usage of the IF diet enhances the emission of adiponectin from adipocytes. There is an opposite association between plasma adiponectin levels and body weight. The Cambuli research regards 104 children with obesity. They contrasted adiponectin's initial concentration with the attention examined after one year of a diet and enhanced physical activity. This concentration was improved by 245%. The increase in adiponectin concentration was comparative to the decrease in body weight. Adiponectin achieves its job by proceeding on adiponectin receptors realized in two isoforms AdipoR1 AdipoR.

It displays anti-atherosclerotic and anti-inflammatory influences by inhibiting the adhesion of monocytes to endothelial cells. It also inhibits the emission of the vascular cell adhesion molecule 1 (VCAM-1), endothelial-leukocyte adhesion molecule 1 (ELAM-1), and intracellular adhesive molecule 1 (ICAM-1) on vascular endothelial cells. The study was proven by Ouchi et al. in in-vitro reports on individuals' aortic endothelial cells incubated for 18 hours in the presence of adiponectin. An adhesion assay assessed adhesion, produced by tumor necrosis element alpha (TNF-alpha), of THP-1-line monocytes to individuals' aortic endothelial cells.

The appearance of the molecules was assessed by ELISA (enzyme-linked immunosorbent assay). The anti-atherosclerotic performance of adiponectin has been proven in several animal models and cell cultures. For example, reports organized by Okamoto et al., using confirmed transcriptase-polymerase chain reaction (real-time) and ELISA testing, explained that adiponectin has an anti-inflammatory action in individual's macrophages by inhibiting the creation of CXC 3 receptor chemokine ligands. In in-vivo reports on mice lacking in apolipoprotein E/adiponectin, there was an enhancement in IP-10in plasma, and enhanced deposition of T lymphocytes vessels and atherosclerosis analyzed to a single apoE deficiency. Matsuda et al. explained in adiponectin-lacking mice that a shortage of this protein enhances smooth muscle cells' propagation and relocation by increasing HB-EGF manifestation (heparin-binding epidermal growth element). The IF diet's link with improved adiponectin amounts was proven in reports organized by Wan et al. These reports were carried out on rats allocated to groups with an ad-lib diet and IF for three months. Animals with an IF diet were destitute of food for 24 hours, every other day. The rats' left coronary artery was ligated to produce myocardial infarction. Animals with an IF diet had a tremendous adiponectin amount, and the area of ischemia was smaller. Moreover, essentially lower inflammatory indexes were examined, while leukocytes and IL6 were analyzed in rats with an ad-lib diet. An essential hormone discharged by adipocytes is leptin. It has a pro-atherogenic influence. Its amount is elevated in obese people and is correlated with body mass index (BMI), total cholesterol, triglycerides, blood pressure, and inflammation markers. These relationships were confirmed in reports sorted out by Sattar et al., in which leptin sums were built up in 550 men with lethal coronary illness (deadly CHD) or nonfatal myocardial localized necrosis (nonfatal MI) and in 1184 patients included in an examination on 5561 British men.

The amount of leptin reduces body weight when using the IF diet. Leptin hyper-action minimizes the danger of atherosclerosis by reducing platelet aggregation and reducing endothelial cell proliferation and migration. Moreover, Resistin plays an essential function in the pathogenesis of atherosclerosis. This mechanism is a cytokine gain from adipocytes, and its amount correlates with resistance to insulin and obesity. It has a proinflammatory action. It also encourages the proinflammatory activity of neutrophils and macrophages and the formation of extracellular deposits in vessels. This way happens by inhibiting AMP-activated protein kinase activation, responsible for the inhibition of neutrophil action. Resistin enhances the appearance of chemotactic monocyte one protein (MCP-1) and SICAM-1in vascular endothelial cells. These examinations were created by Burnett and his team in reports in which they incubated mouse aortic endothelial cells with a recombinant Resistin (adipose tissue-specific secretory factor (ADSF).

Research carried out by Bhutani et al. is proof that the ADF diet display action in modulating adipokines. Consequently, it has cardio-protective and anti-sclerotic influences. The study involved 16 obese people—twelve women and four men. It lasted for ten weeks and involved three phases of nutritive intrusions. The first two weeks were the control phase, the next four weeks involved the ADF diet in which the feeding time was monitored, and the last four weeks were ADF with a self-fed nourishment time by the patient. After eight weeks of using the ADF diet, there was a reduction in leptin amounts associated with reduced body weight and fat content.

The quantity of Resistin was essentially reduced after using the ADF diet, which probably was associated with a reduction in body weight.

Chapter 3
Meal Plan for 14 Days

Meal Plan Week 1

Day	Breakfast	Lunch	Snack
1	Trail mix	Herb-roasted chicken breasts	Squash bites
2	Warm roasted vegetable Farro salad	Zesty Chicken	Zucchini chips
3	Cajun potato, prawn/shrimp, and avocado salad	Chicken quinoa anti-inflammatory	Pepperoni Bites
4	Baked mahi-mahi	Skillet lemon chicken & potatoes with kale	Party meatballs
5	Sheet pan chicken and Brussel sprouts	Grilled chicken salad with mango & avocado	Chicken strips
6	Perfect cauliflower pizza crust	Chicken & snap peas stir fry	Roasted Brussels sprouts with pecans and gorgonzola
7	Sweet potato and black bean burrito	Chicken Caprese sandwich	Artichoke petals bites

Meal Plan Week 2

Day	Breakfast	Lunch	Snack
1	Crockpot black-eyed peas	Zucchini noodles with pesto & chicken	Stuffed beef loin in sticky sauce
2	Peach berry smoothie	Lettuce wraps	Eggplant fries
3	Sweet potato curry with spinach and chickpeas	Grilled chicken breast	Parmesan crisps
4	Poached eggs and avocado toasts	Cheesy chicken salad	Roasted broccoli
5	Sweet potato hash	Chicken breasts with avocado tapenade	Almond flour muffins
6	Blueberry smoothie	Beef & barley soup	Apple bread
7	Almond smoothie	Instant pot chicken	Coconut protein balls

Chapter 4
Intermittent Fasting and Supplements

Not all supplements can provide the health benefits you need. Taking the wrong supplements, especially while you are on intermittent fasting, may bring harm. The right types of health supplements can significantly boost the effects of intermittent fasting.

We will briefly discuss the problems with taking generic supplements, how to choose the right health supplements for those who are into intermittent fasting, and a comprehensive list of health supplements that you should take.

The Problem with Multivitamins

Multivitamins are very popular. Millions of people take multivitamins, and many believe that they are essential in the fight against disease and malnutrition. This is, in fact, a misconception. In reality, not everyone can benefit from multivitamins and instead choose targeted supplements.

Nutritional Imbalance

Many multivitamins contain many specific nutrients such as Vitamin A or C, and not enough of the other essential nutrients such as magnesium. So, there is a tendency to overdose on a few nutrients and not taking enough of the others.

Some manufacturers still include a long list of multivitamins on their labels, but the truth is, some of these vitamins are in very small amounts. Many consumers ignore the insubstantial amounts of important nutrients. How can you fit a range of nutrients in only one pill? Also, we need to consider the nutritional needs of each person. A bodybuilder will require a different set of nutrients compared to a lactating mom.

Low Quality of Multivitamins

Each type of nutrient behaves differently inside the body. While folate is an important B vitamin, folic acid—the form found in generic multivitamins—may increase the risk of colon cancer according to a study published by the University of Chile.

This could be the reason why some researches such as a 2009 study published by the University of East Finland suggest a connection between multivitamins and an increase in mortality, while another research commissioned by the American Medical Association in 2009 reveals no benefit in taking multivitamins.

Furthermore, many multivitamins are manufactured with additives and fillers, which make it difficult for the body to absorb nutrients. Therefore, a minimal amount of important nutrients may reach your cells.

We are actually getting what we pay for with multivitamins. You may convince yourself and choose the generic multivitamins in the store, or you may add a bit and actually choose targeted supplements to help improve your health.

Supplements and Fasting

Eating whole and natural foods are still the best source to get the important nutrients that our body needs. Remember, whole foods may behave differently from their individual components. For example, the nutrients from a piece of broccoli are more accessible compared to consuming an equal amount of nutrients from a powder or a pill.

The antioxidants sourced from natural foods are beneficial, but consuming mega doses of some synthetic antioxidants may come with risks such as the growth of tumors based on a 1993 toxicology research from the University of Hamburg.

Food synergy enables the nutrients in food to work together. Hence, food is more powerful compared to its components. This is why it is crucial to begin with a diet that is rich in nutrients, then add supplements that are based on your goals and needs.

It is important to take note that just because something is natural doesn't mean it is helpful. There is a tendency for some, especially the health buffs, to abuse even food-based vitamins and herbal supplements.

These supplements are still vulnerable to contaminants and heavy metals from manufacturing. Be sure to check the sourcing and quality testing of your supplements. It is ideal to check with a licensed professional who can recommend safe brands of supplements.

Chapter 5
Other Tips to Follow to Make IF More Effective

Find a Worthy Goal

First things first: find a goal that is worth pursuing, or else you will drop the idea at the first sign of resistance. If you don't have a goal that represents a strong ideal, it won't be long before you start telling yourself, "I think I've passed the stage of such childishness." And yes, many women start a new lifestyle change for reasons that they can't keep up when things get tough. For example, the desire to look like models on TV, or social media makes losing weight feel socially acceptable and ok to keep up with trends that can be harmful. These reasons are not enough to keep anyone committed to a full lifestyle change and few wonder why so many people with goals are quick to jump from one lifestyle to another.

Don't go into fasting intermittently because it is the thing to do at the moment. Instead, look for inspiring goals such as:

- Staying fit, young, and healthy.
- Improving your cognitive or brain functions.
- Improving your overall vitality and increase energy levels.

- Balancing hormones, especially during menopausal or post-menopausal stages of life.

- Improving your overall health, thereby increasing longevity.

Do any of these sound good to you? Surely at this stage of your life, you are aware of the inherent risks of doing something merely because others are doing it too. That type of motivation will fail you.

Check Your Hormones

A woman's hormones can be easily thrown out of whack by the slightest change in her already established pattern of behavior. Whether it is a physical change such as altering you're eating pattern or an emotional change such as being irritated or sad, it can bring about hormonal imbalance in a woman even if it is temporary.

But for perimenopausal and menopausal women, hormones can go haywire for reasons even they can't define. She could be feeling really great all week, and without anything changing she could suddenly become fatigued, depressed, and not in the right frame of mind. These changes happen due to the unpredictability of this phase of a woman's life. Because this can happen for no apparent reason, it is best to check your hormonal levels before putting your body through a major lifestyle change. If you've ever had issues with thyroid, cortisol, or adrenal fatigue, ensure that you have these checks before you begin.

This may come as a surprise to some women, but your ovaries produce testosterone too. So, as you grow older and begin to experience a decline in your estrogen and progesterone levels, your testosterone levels are also taking a nosedive. Your libido can be affected by low levels of testosterone and make you feel exhausted and bummed out for no reason at all. Hence, while you are checking your other hormones, don't forget to do a testosterone test. The thyroid and testosterone hormones also help in weight regulation. So, if you intend to shed some weight using intermittent fasting, these tests are very necessary.

Start Slow

To go from having five or six meals daily to eating only once a day can lead to very dire consequences. After confirming that intermittent fasting is suitable for your health, the next thing to do is planning how to ease into the habit. In other words, before you fully implement any intermittent fasting regimen, it is a good practice to first test the waters, so to speak, with a less strict form of fasting. By doing this, it will help your body acclimate to the changes before going into the proper regimen.

Don't Fuss Over What You Can Eat

One common mistake people make when fasting is obsessing over the fasting hours and what to eat when they are finally allowed. Of course, if your fasting window is too small, you are not likely to see any result. Also, don't get too tied up in every little detail of intermittent fasting. For example, you don't have to become too worried because you missed a day. Remember that fasting intermittently should be a lifestyle change if you want to continue to reap the benefits. And for a lifestyle change to be sustainable, you must be able to adapt and use it in a way that even if you face challenges, you will work your way around it somehow. Missing a day or cutting your fast short for reasons beyond your control shouldn't get you worked up and worrying about whether you can do the entire plan. Don't give up.

Again, some people focus too much on what they can eat or not eat. For example, "Can I add just a little butter or cream?" "Would it hurt to eat this type of food during the fasting window?" If your focus is on what you can have or eat while you are fasting, you are giving your attention to the wrong things and putting your mind in an unhelpful state. Give your mind the right focus by concentrating on doing a good, clean, fast, and try to consume only water, tea, or coffee during the window.

Watch Electrolytes

Your body electrolytes are compounds and elements that occur naturally in body fluids, blood, and urine. They can also be ingested through drinks, foods, and supplements. Some of them include magnesium, calcium, potassium, chloride, phosphate, and sodium. Their functions include fluid balance, regulation of the heart and neurological function, acid-base balance, oxygen delivery, and many other functions.

It is important to keep these electrolytes in a state of balance. But many people who practice fasting tend to neglect this and run into problems. Here is a common notion: "Don't let anything into your stomach until the end of your fast" Even those just starting to fast know it doesn't work that way, and they tend to forget or fully stay away from liquids during their fasting window.

When you lose too much water from your body through sweating, vomiting, and diarrhea, or you don't have enough water in your body because you don't drink enough liquids, you increase the risk of electrolyte disorders. It is not okay to drink tea or black coffee throughout the morning period of your fast window. You will wear yourself down if you don't drink enough water. The longer you fast without water, the higher your chances of flushing out electrolytes and running into trouble. You can end up raising your blood pressure, develop muscle twitching and spasms, fatigue, fast heart rate or irregular heartbeat, and many other health problems.

On the other hand, drinking too much water can also tip the water-electrolyte balance. What you want to do is to drink adequate amounts of water and not excess water, whether you are fasting or not.

Give the Calorie Restriction a Rest

Remember that intermittent fasting is different from dieting. Your focus should be on eating healthily during your eating window or eating days instead of focusing on calorie restriction. Even if you are fasting for weight loss, don't obsess over calories. Following a fasting regimen is enough to take care of the calories you consume. It is absolutely unnecessary to engage in a practice that can hurt your metabolism. Combining intermittent fasting with eating too little food in your eating window because you are worried about your calorie intake can cause problems for your metabolism.

One of the major reasons that people push themselves into restricting calories while fasting is their concern for rapid weight loss. You need to be wary of any process that brings about drastic physical changes to your body in very short amounts of time. While it is okay to desire quick results, your health and safety are more important. When you obsess or worry that you are not losing weight as quickly as you want, you are not helping matters. Instead, you are increasing your stress level, and that is counterproductive. You are already taking practical steps toward losing weight by intermittent fasting, why would you want to undo your hard work by unnecessary worrying?

Simply focus on following a sustainable intermittent fasting regimen and let go of the need to restrict your calorie intake. Intermittent fasting will give your body the right number of calories it needs if you do it properly.

The First Meal of the Eating Window Is Key

Breaking your fast is a crucial part of the process because if you don't get it right, it could quickly develop into unhealthy eating patterns. When you break your fast, it is important to have healthy foods around to prevent grabbing unhealthy feel-good snacks. Make sure what you are eating in your window is not a high-sugar or high-carb meal. I recommend that you consider breaking your fast with something that is highly nutrient-dense such as a green smoothie, protein shake, or healthy salad.

As much as possible, avoid breaking your fast with foods from a fast-food restaurant. Eating junk foods after your fast is a quick way to ruin all the hard work you've put in during your fasting window. If, for any reason, you can't prepare your meal, ensure that you order very specific foods that will complement your effort and not destroy what you've built.

Break Your Fast Gently

It is okay to feel very hungry after going for a long time without food, even if you were drinking water all through the fasting window. This is particularly true for people who are just starting with fasting. But don't let the intensity of your hunger push you to eat. You don't want to force food hurriedly into your stomach after going long without food or you might hurt yourself and experience stomach distress. Take it slow when you break your fast. Eat light meals in small portions first when you break your fast. Wait for a couple of minutes for your stomach to get used to the presence of food again before continuing with a normal-sized meal.

The waiting period will douse any hunger pangs and remove the urge to rush your meal. For example, break your fast with a small serving of salad and wait for about 15 minutes. Drink some water and then after about five more minutes, you can eat a normal-sized meal.

Nutrition Is Important

Although intermittent fasting is not dieting and so, does not specify which foods to eat, limit, and completely avoid, it makes sense to eat healthily. This means focusing on eating a balanced diet, such as:

- Whole grains.

- Fruits and vegetables (canned in water, fresh, or frozen).

- Lean sources of protein (lentils, beans, eggs, poultry, tofu, and so on).

- Healthy fats (nuts, seeds, coconuts, avocados, olive oil, olive, and fatty fish).

It simply doesn't make any sense to go for 16 hours (or more) without food and then spend the rest of the day eating junk. Even if you follow the 5:2 diet and limit your calorie intake to only 500 calories per day for two days, it is totally illogical to follow it with five days of eating highly processed foods and low-quality meals. Combining intermittent fasting with unbalanced diets will lead to nutritional deficiencies and defeat the goal of fasting in the first place. Realize that intermittent fasting is not a magic wand that makes all poor eating habits vanish in a poof! For the practice to work, you must be deliberate about the types of food you eat.

Chapter 6. The Intermittent Fasting Type

16/8 Method

This is just about the most popular fasting method since it's so schedule-based, meaning there are no surprises. This will give you the freedom to control when you eat based on the everyday life of yours. The sixteen is the number of hours you're likely to be fasting, which may also be lowered to twelve or perhaps fourteen hours if that fits into your life better. Then you're eating period is going to be between eight and ten hours every day. This might seem daunting, but it just means that you are skipping an entire meal. Many people choose to begin their fast around 7 or 8 p.m. and then do not eat until 11 or noon the next day, which means they fast for the recommended 16 hours. Of course, it isn't as bad as it sounds since they are sleeping during this time, so what it comes down to is eating dinner and then not eating again the next day around lunch, so you are just skipping breakfast.

You will be doing it every day, so finding the hours that work for you are important. If you work the third shift, then switching you're eating period around to fit into your schedule is important. If you find yourself being run down and sluggish, tweak your fasting hours until you find a healthy balance. Granted, there will be some adjustment, because, chances are, your body is not accustomed to skipping entire meals.

However, this should go away after a couple of weeks, and if it doesn't then try starting your fasting period earlier in the day allowing you to eat earlier the next, or alter it however you need to feel healthy and happy.

Lean-Gains Method (14:10)

The lean-gains method has several different incarnations on the web, but its fame comes from the fact that it helps shed fat while building it into muscle almost immediately. Through the lean-gains method, you'll find yourself able to shift all that fat to be muscle through a rigorous practice of fasting, eating right, and exercising.

Through this method, you fast anywhere from 14 to 16 hours and spend the remaining 10 or 8 hours each day engaged in eating and exercise. As opposed to the crescendo, this method features daily fasting and eating, rather than alternated days of eating versus not. Therefore, you don't have to be quite cautious about extending the physical effort to exercise on the days you are fasting because those days when you're fasting are every day!

For the lean-gaining method, start fasting only for 14 hours and work it up to 16 if you feel comfortable with it, but never forget to drink enough water and be careful about spending too much energy on exercise! Remember that you want to grow in health and potential through intermittent fasting. You'll certainly not want to lose any of that growth by forcing the process along.

20:4 Method

Stepping things up a notch from the 14:10 and 16:8 methods, the 20:4 method is a tough one to master, for it is rather unforgiving. People talk about this method of intermittent fasting as intense and highly restrictive. Still, they also say that the effects of living this method are almost unparalleled with all other tactics.

For the 20:4 method, you'll fast for 20 hours each day and squeeze all your meals, all your eating, and all your snacking into 4 hours. People who attempt 20:4 normally have two smaller meals or just one large meal and a few snacks during their 4-hour window to eat, and it is up to the individual which four hours of the day they devote to eating.

The trick for this method is to make sure you're not overeating or bingeing during those 4-hour windows to eat. It is all-too-easy to get hungry during the 20-hour fast and have that feeling then propel you into intense and unrealistic hunger or meal sizes after the fast period is over. Be careful if you try this method. If you're new to intermittent fasting, work your way up to this one gradually, and if you're working your way up already, only make the shift to 20:4 when you know you're ready. It would surely disappoint if all your progress with intermittent fasting got hijacked by one poorly thought-out goal with the 20:4 method.

Meal Skipping

Meal skipping is an extremely flexible form of intermittent fasting that can provide all of the benefits of intermittent fasting but with less strict scheduling. If you are not someone who has a typical schedule or feels like a stricter variation of the intermittent fasting diet will serve you, meal skipping is a viable alternative.

Many people who choose to use meal skipping find it a great way to listen to their bodies and follow their basic instincts. If they are not hungry, they simply don't eat that meal. Instead, they wait for the next one. Meal skipping can also help people who have time constraints and who may not always be able to get in a certain meal of the day.

It is important to realize that with meal skipping, you may not always be maintaining a 10- 16-hour window of fasting. As a result, you may not get every benefit that comes from other fasting diets. However, this may be a great solution for people who want an intermittent fasting diet that feels more natural. It may also be a great idea for those looking to begin listening to their bodies more so that they can adjust to a more intense variation of the diet with greater ease. It can be a great transitional diet for you if you are not ready to jump into one of the other fasting diets just yet.

Warrior Diet Fasting

The most extreme form of intermittent fasting is known as the warrior diet. This intermittent fasting cycle follows a 20-hour fasting window with a short 4-hour eating window. During that eating window, individuals are supposed to only consume raw fruits and vegetables. They can also eat one large meal. Typically, the eating window occurs at night time so people can snack throughout the evening, have a large meal, and then resume fasting.

Because of the length of fasting taking place during the warrior diet, people should also consume a fairly hearty level of healthy fats. Doing so will give the body something to consume during the fast to produce energy with. A small number of carbohydrates can also be incorporated to support energy levels, too.

People who eat the warrior diet tend to believe that humans are natural nocturnal eaters and that we are not meant to eat throughout the day. The belief is that eating this way follows our natural circadian rhythms, allowing our body to work optimally.

The only people who should consider doing the warrior diet are those who have already had success with other forms of intermittent fasting and who are used to it. Attempting to jump straight into the warrior diet can have serious repercussions for anyone who is not used to intermittent fasting. Even still, those who are used to it may find this particular style too extreme for them to maintain.

Eat-Stop-Eat (24 Hour) Method

This method of fasting is incredibly similar to the crescendo method. The only discernable difference is that there's no anticipation of increasing into a more intense fasting pattern with time. For the eat-stop-eat method, you decide which days you want to take off from eating, and then you run with it until you've lost that weight and then you keep running with the lifestyle for good because you won't be able to imagine life without it.

The eat-stop-eat method involves one to two days a week being 100% oriented towards fasting, with the other five to six days concerning "business as normal." The one or two days spent fasting are then full 24-hour days spent without eating anything at all. These days, of course, water and coffee are still fine to drink, but no food items can be consumed whatsoever. Exercise is also frowned upon on those fasting days, but see what your body can handle before you decide how that should all work out.

Some people might start thinking they're using the crescendo method but end up sticking with eat-stop-eat.

Alternate-Day Method

The alternate-day method is admittedly a little confusing, but the reason it could be so confusing could come, in part, from how much wiggle room it provides for the practitioner. This method is great for people who don't have a consistent schedule or any sense of one, it is incredibly forgiving for those who don't quite have everything together for themselves yet.

When it comes down to it, alternate-day intermittent fasting is really up to you. You should try to fast every other day, but it doesn't have to be that precise. Similarly, with the crescendo method, as long as you fast two to three days a week, with a break day or two in between each fasting day, you're set! Then, you'll want to eat normally for three or four days out of each week, and when you encounter a fasting day, you don't even need to completely fast!

Alternate-day fasting is a solid place to start from, especially if you work a varying schedule or still have yet to get used to a consistent one. If you want to make things more intense from this starting point, the alternate-day method can easily become the eat-stop-eat method, the crescendo method, or the 5:2 method. Essentially, this method is a great place to begin.

12:12 Method

As another of the more natural ways of intermittent fasting, the 12:12 approach is well-suited to beginning practitioners. Many people live out the 12:12 method without any forethought simply because of their sleeping and eating schedule, but turning 12:12 into a conscious practice can have just as many positive effects on your life as the more drastic 20:4 method claims.

According to a study conducted in the University of Alabama, for this method, in particular, you fast for 12 hours and then enter a 12-hour eating window. It's not difficult whatsoever to get three small meals and several snacks, or two big meals and a snack into your day with this method. With 12:12, the standard meal timing works just fine.

Ultimately, this method is a great one to start from, for a lot of variation can be built into this scheduling when you're ready to make things more interesting. Effortlessly and without much effort, 12:12 can become 14:10 or even 16:8, and in seemingly no time, you can find yourself trying alternate-day or crescendo methods, too. Start with what's normal for you, and this method might be exactly that!

Chapter 7
How to Plan

Life Fasting Tracker

Utilize your cell phone to set updates for yourself of when to eat, what to eat, and when your fast days are. It works well when utilizing it to set updates for when you should drink water, especially for the individuals who think it's difficult to keep track of water and other essential nutrients.

Making a Change

You have to keep in mind that intermittent fasting isn't an eating routine; it is a way of life, an eating plan that you are in charge of, and one that is not difficult to achieve. Before you know it, fasting will turn out to be natural.

When to Start

Start today, not tomorrow, or after a specific occasion or gathering. Select the suitable fast feasible for you, and start with it right away. Never hold off until a particular day; when you start, you will acquire energy and it will become important for your day, in the same way as other things are your priorities.

Measure What You're Eating

Just to lessen your burden, try to reduce your meal 3 days before you fast; it is smart to start to decrease the amount of food you are eating or dish up less. This causes your body to start to get used to the possibility that it doesn't need a bowl full of food when you're fasting.

Keep Up Your Exercise Plan

If you already exercise, that's great, you don't need to change it. You can follow the exercise routine that suits you. If you don't usually exercise daily, start doing it immediately. Make a plan for yourself and gradually increase your walking, running, and jogging interval the next day, increase it in 10 to 15 minutes to whatever suits you.

Do Your Research

Read about intermittent fasting from other sources. Talk to your friends or people around you. You might find someone who can share their practical experience of intermittent fasting. Try to find authentic tried and tested. That way, you won't be stuck in the middle, not knowing what to eat and what to avoid.

Have Fun

Ultimately, have a good time and see what your body can do, much more than 50. It is imperative to realize that because you are a specific age doesn't mean you are unequipped for seeking another way of life change. Praise yourself when it is required, track your development, change where the need is, and get good sleep. Do not overburden yourself; just be consistent.

Know Your BMI

The Body Mass Index (BMI) is calculated by dividing a person's weight in kilograms by their height in meters squared. A high BMI can indicate obesity, and a low BMI indicates low body fat or being underweight. The BMI can be used to test for weight categories that could lead to health issues, but it does not signify an individual's body fatness or health. There is a certain constant scale on which BMI is considered normal, high, and low.

How to Calculate Your BMI?

To determine your BMI, compare your weight (lbs.) x 703 divided by your height (in). Whenever you have determined your BMI, you can contrast it with the weight file outline to figure out which classification you are classed into.

BMI	Weight Status
Below 18.5	Underweight
18.5-24.9	The healthy or normal weight
25.0-29.9	Overweight
30.0 and above	Obese

Chapter 8
Diet in Menopause

Here are some remedies for symptoms that are common among women in their forties and fifties. Remember, any questions you have should always be discussed with your healthcare provider first. Other medications or potentially adverse side effects can be available. It would help if you decided the choices are better for you as a couple.

Mood Changes

Hormone fluctuations during perimenopause can leave some women feeling out of control. Increased irritability, anxiety, exhaustion, and depressed moods are common complaints. Relaxation and stress-reduction strategies, such as deep-breathing exercises and massage, as well as a healthy lifestyle (including good diet and physical exercise) and fun, self-nurturing activities, can all be beneficial. Some people use over-the-counter remedies like St. John's wort or vitamin B6 to alleviate menopause symptoms.

Discussing your mood problems with your doctor will help you figure out what's causing them, check for serious depression, and decide on the best course of action. Prescription antidepressant drugs can be prescribed for depression to remedy a chemical imbalance. While it takes many weeks to feel the full effect of one of these treatments, several women report significant improvements with very few side effects. Hot flashes have been shown to be treated by certain antidepressants. When antidepressant treatment is combined with counseling or psychotherapy, it is most effective.

Urinary Incontinence

Although urinary incontinence is described as the involuntary loss of urine over time, most women would describe it as an unfortunate, unexpected, and unwanted nuisance. Fortunately, there are non-surgical and non-medication methods for treating different types of incontinence. To keep urine filtered (clear and pale yellow), drink plenty of water and avoid foods or drinks rich in acid or caffeine, which can irritate the bladder lining. Grapefruit, bananas, tomatoes, coffee, and caffeine-containing soft drinks are among them.

Having a Hard Time Falling Asleep

Establish a consistent sleep schedule and routine:

- Even on weekends, get up and go to bed at the same times every day.

- Before going to bed, unwind and relax by reading a book, listening to music, or taking a long bath.

- Tryptophan is found in milk and peanuts, and it helps the body relax.

- A cup of chamomile tea could also help.

- Maintain a comfortable amount of light, noise, and temperature in your bedroom—dark, quiet, and cool are conducive to sleep.

- Use the bedroom for sleeping and sex.

- Avoid caffeine and alcohol.

Sexual Dissatisfaction

Menopause causes changes in sexual function by reducing ovarian hormone output, which can cause vaginal dryness and a decline in sexual function. To combat these changes, try the following:

Vaginal lubricants: these drugs, which are available without a prescription, reduce pressure and make intercourse easier when the vagina is dry. Since oil-based products like Vaseline can irritate the skin, only water-soluble products should be used. Just use vaginal products; avoid hand creams and lotions that contain alcohol or perfumes, as well as warming/tingling and flavored lubricants that may irritate sensitive tissue. (Astroglide, Moist Again, and Silk-E are some of the vaginal lubricants available.)

Vaginal moisturizers: these items, which are often available without a prescription, help people with moderate vaginal atrophy preserve or increase vaginal moisture (when tissues of the vulva and the lining of the vagina become thin, dry, less elastic, and less lubricated as a result of estrogen loss). They also keep the pH of the vaginal environment low, ensuring a safe vaginal environment.

Replens and K-Y Long-lasting Vaginal Moisturizer are two examples.) These drugs are more long-lasting than vaginal lubricants and can be used on a regular basis.

Last but not least, women can maintain vaginal health by engaging in painless sexual activity on a regular basis, which increases blood flow to the genital region.

Menopause Natural Treatments That Actually Work

Women who do not want to use hormone therapy to relieve menopausal symptoms have a number of effective alternatives. For memory issues, weight gain, high cholesterol, and vaginal symptoms, here are some natural lifestyle tips:

Natural Remedies: A Word of Caution

Always keep in mind that normally does not imply risk-free. Many herbal, fruit and dietary supplements may interfere with prescription drugs or worsen chronic medical conditions. Natural methods are not without risk, and the more you know, the better equipped you will be to select therapies that will keep you healthy and secure.

Check with your medical professional before choosing to use alternative and complementary treatments for your menopause symptoms, and read up on any potential side effects and cautions for any remedy you're considering.

Memory Problems

It's aggravating to try to remember a word or name that's on the tip of your tongue but you can't get it out. As you prepare to leave the house, forgetting where you put your car keys or where you put your glasses will drive you insane. Does this ring a bell? When they approach perimenopause, many women begin to notice memory problems.

Green tea consumption has been linked to a number of health benefits, including immune system enhancement and cancer prevention. Green tea is now being linked to preventing memory-damaging enzyme activity in studies. It has a small number of side effects and is widely available.

A sufficient amount of sleep is needed for your brain to process memory tasks. Both short and longer naps seem to help memory work, according to research. If you can't get a cat nap during the day, make sure you get enough overnight sleep to avoid memory issues.

Control of Stress

Stress is a big memory sapper. Pay attention to your stress level, whether you're having trouble focusing or recalling everyday things. Even short-term stress has been shown to affect learning and memory, according to research. Divorce, illness, raising children, and elderly parents are only a few of the issues that can arise during the menopause process. It is a survival skill to take care of yourself and reduce tension in your life. Memory issues may be an early warning sign that the stress level is rising.

Weight Gain

For women over 50, weight gain is often a source of irritation. The exact mechanism by which estrogen affects metabolism is unknown. What is apparent, however, is that many women who have never struggled to maintain a healthy weight before menopause continue to do so during and after the menopause era. Although there are no validated herbal weight loss remedies, there are lifestyle and dietary improvements that can help you naturally reduce your weight gain.

Stress Management

Stress, especially the production of the stress hormone cortisol, may impair your body's ability to maintain a healthy weight. It would be easier for your body to regulate calories and fat metabolism if you keep cortisol levels down.

Diet Must-Haves

Menopause is an excellent time to assess your diet and make lifestyle changes that will benefit you for the rest of your life. It would help if you amended your thinking to include a good menopause diet that will set the stage for balanced post-menopause as your metabolism slows and you begin to treat calories differently.

Exercise

Everyone agrees that exercise is beneficial to one's health. However, when you approach menopause, it becomes an essential part of the overall health strategy. Weight loss, of course, necessitates increased physical activity. Exercise, on the other hand, is an all-purpose solution to menopause wellbeing since it improves memory, mood, and bone health. Exercise is the only thing that can help you control your weight to its full potential.

Sleep

You would think that getting enough sleep would sabotage your weight loss efforts, but the opposite is true. When you don't get enough sleep, it makes you want to eat more and causes your body to store fat around your midsection. A good night's sleep helps the body reset and recover from the pressures of the day. If you get enough sleep, the body can function more effectively in any way.

Cholesterol Levels Are High

As estrogen levels drop during menopause, your cholesterol levels will rise. Women are soon at the same risk as men for heart disease. You can lower cholesterol levels in a number of natural ways.

Soy and Red Clover

Soy protein has been shown to lower "bad" (LDL) cholesterol and lower total cholesterol levels. Red clover appears to increase "good" (HDL) cholesterol while lowering triglycerides. These plant estrogens may step in to protect your heart when your own estrogen levels drop.

Whole Grain Oats

Including whole grain oats in your diet will reduce total and LDL cholesterol levels, lowering cardiac risk.

Melatonin

Melatonin can help raise HDL cholesterol levels without increasing overall cholesterol levels, in addition to assisting with sleep. This may be beneficial for women who have a higher risk of heart disease. If you're taking melatonin for sleep, you might notice that it lowers your cholesterol as a side effect.

Symptoms of the Vaginal Canal

Two concerns that women may have difficulty getting to their doctors are the loss of satisfaction during sexual intercourse and the beginning of urine leakage. There are a few things you can do if you're getting vaginal symptoms as you approach menopause:

Wild Yam Cream

Creams made from wild yam contain a phytoestrogen that, like other estrogen creams, can help relieve symptoms locally.

Vitamin E and Flaxseed Oil

Whether taken orally or applied directly to the vagina, the combination of vitamin E and flaxseed oil may provide some relief from vaginal and urinary symptoms. Women usually take them as oral supplements, but creams containing them may also be applied directly to the vaginal region.

Vaginal Moisturizers and Lubricants

Vaginal moisturizers operate for many days to make the vagina more elastic, and vaginal lubricants help minimize friction and pain throughout intercourse. Water-based products are less likely to cause an allergic reaction and are widely available in pharmacies.

Chapter 9. Myths About Intermittent Fasting

Now that we have seen some intermittent fasting types and chosen which method suits us the most, the next step would be to rid our minds of certain myths that people have initiated about intermittent fasting over the years. One credible characteristic of the human mouth and hands is their ability to talk and write critically. People would always have a different view and not flow in synergy with what is brought to the table irrespective of how prospect-filled it may appear. Certain myths have come up over the years about the concept of intermittent fasting and it would only be to have me address this in this book. Here are a few:

Intermittent Fasting Is a Road to Starvation

A little enlightenment on this would be in order. Starvation is a condition where someone suffers severely due to a lack of food. It is wrong to think that not eating for 24 to 48 hours starves the body. Research has inadvertently shown that for the body to get started and experience a reduction in metabolic rate, an individual has to not eat for over 60 hours. That is almost three days. As individuals, tight work schedules prevent us from eating for a more significant part of the day and even though we expend a lot of energy doing our work, we still do not break down.

The Burden of Hunger

Some others say that you will feel hungry all day long while doing intermittent fasting. The human body is very adaptive. That is why impoverished or poor individuals can stay for almost a day without food. They are healthy and working tirelessly. From the second week of intermittent fasting, hunger gets low; your body adjusts to your new routine. Just as your body adjusts when saddled with more energy-consuming activities. Here's another thing: most times we are most likely to feel hungry easily when we are in an idle state (doing nothing). Something else you could do is to keep yourself busy all the while during your fasting periods. Getting busy takes our minds away from a lot of things including food, we're fully focused on what we have at hand.

Eating Frequently Boosts Your Metabolism

Now it is another myth generally acknowledged by many people that eating often boosts metabolism. We cannot deny that calories are expended in metabolic processes; this is very true. This is also seen in the digestion of food and known as the Thermic Effect of Food. The body uses about 10% of your overall calorie intake to do this. On the other hand, now, here's where this myth is faulting. What matters is not how frequently you eat, but the number of calories you eat. Now someone consuming six diets of about 500 calories is the same as consuming three diets containing a thousand calories. Therefore, this is the wrong myth.

Dietary Glucose for the Brain

Here's another common misconception. Some people believe that if you do not eat carbs every once in a while, your brain will cease to function. The reason for this is that the brain uses glucose as its only source of fuel. On the other hand, this myth is faulted too because of the concept of gluconeogenesis. This is a process whereby the body synthesizes glucose from non-carbohydrate sources. During long fasts, such as this and low-carb dieting, your body can produce ketone bodies from dietary fats. These ketone bodies feed a part of the brain until it significantly reduces its glucose requirements.

Reduction in Muscle Mass

People have also concluded that intermittent fasting reduces body mass. Although this sometimes happens during fasting, any experiment hasn't proved that it happens more with intermittent fasting than other fast forms. Recent studies show a significant increase in muscle mass for individuals who consume all the calorie requirement in one big meal in a day. It is a predominant technique among bodybuilders, it maintains the muscles. It enhances a considerable amount of weight loss with minimal reduction in muscle mass. This myth is flawed as much evidence proves that intermittent fasts have minimal effect on muscle mass.

Incessant Eating Ensures Good Health

People think that when they eat incessantly, they make good health. This is not entirely true. The body indeed requires nutrients and energy to thrive. Still, cellular repair processes are engaged during intermittent fast periods. This cellular repair process known as autophagy uses dysfunctional and waste proteins for energy. It also prevents aging, cancer and Alzheimer's disease. Some studies have shown that snacking and eating regularly most times harm your body in different ways. For example, when you take a diet with many calories, you cause your liver to become fatty, making you more likely to get fatty liver disease.

Additionally, some research has come up to say that you put yourself more in danger of colorectal cancer if you eat often. Therefore, this further proves that intermittent fast has more health and metabolic benefits than you could imagine.

Skipping Breakfast Can Make You Fat

I also don't know how this myth came about or how it came to be believed. Well, that is how myths are. It is thought that skipping breakfast increases your meal cravings, thus making you consume more food. However, research has proven that skipping breakfast does not have any signs of individuals' weight gain or otherwise. Therefore, you must pay attention to your specific needs. Breakfast is a must for some people and some others can do without it.

Indiscipline Eating Habits on Work Days

Now you engaging in intermittent fasting does not give you the leverage to be glut tonic and eat whatever comes to the eyes. In as much as intermittent fasting helps burn up a lot of calories, replacing the burnt-up calories with even more significant amounts on fast off days counters productive results. It's like shooting yourself on the leg. You take away a piece of dirt and bring in a basket full. At all times, a healthy eating habit should be maintained. Adequate and healthy calorie consumption should be checked and monitored. This is why it is mostly advised that you begin intermittent fasts with a dietician/doctor's assistance. Do not pull down your longhouse of cards with your own hands; self-discipline is a principal element that can help.

Intermittent Fasting Is Never Ending

Here's another myth. Some people have themselves and others believe that once you begin an intermittent fast, you have to keep it going for life. Now to these sets of people, I would love to ask the straightforward question: What was the purpose of the fast in the first place? To burn up a lot of calories and mostly achieve weight loss, not so? Now this eating plan being effective is seeing that the desired result has been achieved. Once the desired results have been seen, there is no need to continue with the exercise. All you need to do from then is watch what you eat, so you won't get excessive calories stored up again. Intermittent fasting helps you train your taste buds to loathe foods with a high percentage of calories; you don't have to struggle to abstain from them anymore after staying through to the intermittent fasting plan for you.

These myths do not clamp down the efficacy of the intermittent fasting method. Logically and ideally, intermittent fasting has more health and metabolic benefits than can be seen. Maybe they just choose to ignore the positives and center on the negatives. The benefits of intermittent fasting even over very short terms cannot be over-emphasized. Fasting exposes the body to a lot of beneficial processes that bulky calories would not let it access. Gene expressions, metabolic waste removal processes, the formation of new neurons and cellular repair are some of these beneficial processes that go on in the body during fasting to mention, but a few.

Chapter 10
Common Mistakes

Searching for an Excessive Number of Improvements Too Fast

You are planning to start something new and you are anxious to get all the awards as fast as anyone might think possible. It is simply normal that you are amped up for this new way of life and you need to completely jump into it. By the by, endeavoring to quickly get a particular number of enhancements too soon may disturb your undertakings.

The key is to start step by step with a few changes in a steady progression. For example, in the event that you have decided to do two 500-calorie days consistently while having an ordinary measure of calories the other 5, think about starting with just one single 500-calorie day. After a long time, you will feel surer including the second day into your week after week plan.

Not Taking Care of Your Hydration

Remaining in a fasting state can be testing whether or not you are not eating. Most beverages will break the fast and exceptionally decrease any advantages. Notwithstanding, the way that they are fat and calorie-free it is definitely not keen to drink "diet" soda pops. Undoubtedly, even sugars that have 0 calories can contrarily impact your insulin levels.

Mistaking Thirst for Hunger

While it is critical not to drink wrong liquids when fasting, it is comparably fundamental to guarantee you drink enough water. Not getting enough water can make you hungry, and it is definitely not hard to now and then mistake hunger for hunger.

Individuals get a lot of water from a decent piece of the food sources they eat. Overall food information expresses that 20% of the water our bodies use starts from food. This suggests that on the off chance that you are not eating for a couple of hours you should drink around 20% more water than expected to make up for any shortage.

Eating Unhealthy Foods

Since intermittent fasting isn't for the most part a diet plan, there are no food sources that are "illegal." This can lead numerous individuals to fall into the catch of gorge on shoddy nourishment the second their fasting is up and the eating time opens. Do whatever it takes not to make a propensity for unfortunate eating imagining that fasting will make up for it.

Cause a summary of the multitude of solid food sources you to do appreciate. Do customary looking for food and attempt to adhere to your food choices. While satisfying your craving with not actually solid bites here and there can be okay, for ideal well-being and weight reduction accomplishment, it is critical to eat as healthy as conceivable in light of the current situation. Eating the correct nourishment is essential to exploiting any weight-reduction plan. Nourishments plentiful in calcium, protein, and nutrient B-12 ought to be high on your staple rundown, especially for ladies more than 50.

Indulging After Each Fast

This is probably the best snare for the 2 novices and individuals who have been fasting intermittently for a long time. Rehearsing intermittent fasting to get more fit will lose viability in the event that you wind up taking in an exorbitant measure of calories on each possibility you need to eat.

One way to deal with keep away from indulging is to eat bigger measures of better nourishments during your eating window. This would incorporate loads of solid plates of blended greens and fresh vegetables. It is also a shrewd plan to orchestrate meals and having flavors arranged before your fast period begins. Subsequently, you are not enticed to simply get anything. Recollect that it can take as long as around 14 days until you have changed and adjusted to the point that you won't feel that ravenous after each fasting period.

Attempting to Stick to the Wrong Plan

There is a wide range of ways to deal with put intermittent fasting into your day-by-day plan. For example, if your fasting plan incorporates not eating from 8 p.m. until early evening each day and you have a difficult action that starts directly in the initial segment of the day, this is in all probability not the right arrangement for you.

What works for one individual may not really fit in for another. To get the most prizes of intermittent fasting, you should take as much time as is needed to altogether investigate various sorts of plans. It is ok in the event that it takes somewhat more to discover the arrangement that best works for you.

Working Out Too Much or Too Little

It is basic to stay as unique as could be expected, yet you would not really like to exaggerate, particularly during your fasting times. A couple of novices may feel overpowered, starting to follow another eating plan, and may neglect practice through and through. Others may be excited to the point that they wind up trying too hard.

It is a keen idea to pick a moderate exercise plan, especially when starting. Walking the pooch for 20 minutes or riding your bike to work are basic ways to deal with add moderate exercise to your standard schedule.

Not Drinking Enough Water

Perhaps, the most widely recognized and effectively avoidable intermittent fasting botches is not to take in enough water. We realize that drinking water is principal for general well-being, obviously, yet it is much more critical when you are fasting. Why? Since more often than not when we feel hungry, we are really dried out.

Would you be able to envision how your appetite may be impacted by the absence of water when you are attempting to experience the fundamental piece of the day without eating? Sneaking more water into your day is just about as straightforward as several fundamental changes. A couple of individuals are really exhausted from drinking plain water. Trust me, one thing that might be a good thought is 2 to 3 Mio Drops (or other water enhancers) to water. It will have a colossal impact!

Misconstruing Real Hunger Signs

Maybe the best thing that I have gained from my intermittent fasting test is that I found a decent speed about when hunger shows. It doesn't come at 9 a.m., the point at which I have been wakeful for 1 hour and last ate a late-night snack at 11 p.m. the earlier evening.

However, once more, you are not actually ravenous. Intermittent fasting will instruct you that on the off potential for success that you have by fasting sufficiently long, as a rule, your "hunger" will obscure commonly in close to 5 to 10 minutes. It, in all likelihood, previously occurred without you seeing or giving it a specific idea.

How often grinding away you were wanting to go to eat, at that point a few nonetheless, some very late surge work appeared, and 1 or 2 hours cruised by, while you ignored your stomach's dissent? What before resembled the direst need, eating, was dominated by something new that sprung up. What's more, you endure!

Regardless, yielding and eating too soon is one of the genuine misunderstandings with intermittent fasting. Feel that essentially drinking some water and permitting it ten minutes or somewhere in the vicinity, you will, for the most part, your hunger will quiet down. Make an effort not to break your intermittent fasting plan before you even start. Do whatever it takes not to effectively yield to false yearning!

Blaming Intermittent Fasting to Overeat

Quite possibly, the most unsafe intermittent fasting botches is yield to the impulse to say, "What the hell, I have starved myself all through all the day, I have the right to remunerate myself for dinner!" and afterward making a plunge an insane dining experience of shoddy nourishment bombarding yourself with unfortunate stuff. Kindly, don't be that lady. You would feel miserable and probably put on weight, and we don't need that.

Notwithstanding, the way that intermittent fasting isn't a diet since it doesn't restrict what you eat, it is yet basic to make better food choices. You need a large portion of all to have a healthy connection with your food and your body. You can totally gorge and put on weight even by eating just once each day, on the off chance that you are eating a more prominent number of calories than your body burns through.

Not Eating Enough

In the event that you presently can't seem to endeavor intermittent fasting, the danger of not eating enough during eating times may seem, by all accounts, to be nonsensical. All things considered, for certain individuals, not eating for an especially significant period is not bizarre to turn out to be less ravenous.

Now and again, fasting can completely execute your craving. Except if you are intentionally doing an absolute fast (not proposed if not under clinical control). Nonetheless, it is definitely not rather a smart thought to choose not to eat enough. On the off chance that you ought not to eat adequately for a really long time, you can undoubtedly wreck your assimilation and unbalance your chemicals. Besides, you will keep your body from getting principal supplements, which can help your well-being evading issues that are undeniably more significant than passing several extra pounds. Counsel your doctor about a total, sound calorie consumption that is good for weight reduction and may help you arrive at your ideal results.

Neglecting to Plan Your Meals in Advance

While calorie counting isn't significant (anyway genuinely, you will give more indications of progress results in the event that you do it), cautiously arranging and pondering what you will eat when you're eating period shows up is an incredible intermittent fasting hack. This will permit you not to need to extemporize when you are at long last going to take a seat at the table.

As opposed to going like "I'm starving and need to eat now regardless" and afterward making a beeline for the nearest, least expensive, and more unfortunate shoddy nourishment, you better figure out how to advise yourself "Indeed, I'm feeling hungry now, yet I can pause, I'm not kicking the bucket and something solid and delectable is hanging tight for me, later."

Using this chance to consider what you will eat, when you eat, and adhering to better choices will just have benefits for you over the long haul. You will figure out how to eat for compelling weight reduction, while diminishing caloric admission, keeping you fulfilled, and boosting your fearlessness. In the event that you are fasting for 16 hours, you can undoubtedly contribute 5 minutes of your opportunity to arrange for what meal will break your fast later.

Not Exercising at All

While the facts confirm that you really could, regardless, lose a great deal of weight with intermittent fasting even without working out by any means, why in the world would you leave behind the amazing opportunity to lose fundamentally more, faster, and with a lot of different advantages for your well-being? It truly has absolutely no explanation. Time can't avoid being time. A month is a month. If in 1 month you could be sluggish and shed 5 pounds or exercise 3 times each week and lose 10, wouldn't you go for the 10?

Chapter 11
Intermittent Fasting and Exercise

Working out while intermittent fasting can be a little complicated, but there are ways to make it easier. Women over 50 years old may want to incorporate exercise with intermittent fasting. What's the best way for women over 50 to combine exercise with intermittent fasting? The key is not to overeat after working out. It is unnecessary to eat as soon as you finish exercising, wait at least a couple of hours and then make your meal small and light. For example, if you have worked out in the morning, wait until about noon or later for your meal and include some protein and vegetables in it. You may want to avoid eating too many fibrous foods that can cause digestive issues such as gas or bloating during a workout session. It is possible to do intermittent fasting without exercise, but the combination is especially beneficial for women over 50 years old. This will help you lose weight and keep it off, especially if you incorporate exercise with intermittent fasting on a regular basis.

Walking or hiking is a great way to get some exercise while only eating one meal a day. These activities should be done for at least 30 minutes to burn fat and keep the weight off effectively. (36 calories per mile for walking).

When you combine intermittent fasting with exercise, the benefits can be substantial. Intermittent fasting will help you lose weight by burning more fat. It can also help you get leaner if you combine exercise with intermittent fasting on a regular basis because it will keep your metabolism up and burn even more calories. There are many reports of women doing intermittent fasting and exercising regularly and losing several pounds in just a short period.

When you fast, there are no negative side effects that interfere with your workout program such as other fad diets cause. With intermittent fasting, you can eat throughout the day and not have to worry about it interfering with your workouts.

Cardio

Cardio exercise has numerous benefits, but for women over the age of 50, there are a few that are particularly beneficial. Women over 50 years old who do cardio exercise can improve their cholesterol levels. When you burn fat while doing cardio, it is released into the bloodstream where it attaches to certain proteins called apoproteins and then is taken back out of the bloodstream into the liver where it is used as an energy source for the body. This can help your cholesterol levels if you do cardio exercise and intermittent fasting.

Cardio exercise helps reduce the risk of heart disease and stroke. When women over 50 years old do cardio exercise, it keeps their cardiovascular system strong, which will help prevent heart disease and stroke. Women over 50 years old who have a healthy lifestyle can play an important role in preventing heart disease and stroke.

Cardio Exercise 1: Jumping

When you jump with your whole body, your muscles work harder as they are used to stress, resulting in a higher metabolism. As you move your body more frequently during the day during cardio exercises such as running or walking, your muscles will become stronger and more toned. You can work up to doing cardio exercise for 30 minutes, several times per week.

Cardio Exercise 2: Running/Jogging

Running or jogging is one of the best cardio exercises and is excellent for women over 50 years old who do no other kinds of exercise. Running or jogging may not be necessary for younger women who are only in their 20s and 30s, but if you are over 50 years old it is a great way to keep your body fit and healthy. You can increase the amount of time you run depending upon how much time you have available due to the work schedule or other responsibilities that need to be met. It is very important for women over 50 years old to stay active and exercise. If you don't, your body will begin to shut down faster. You need to do cardio exercise 2 to 3 times per week for optimal results.

Combining cardio exercise with intermittent fasting, particularly in the morning hours, will help you lose weight and keep it off because the combination causes your body to burn more fat. The fat burned by the combination is typically not stored elsewhere, but rather is released into your bloodstream, where it attaches to various proteins and is then removed from your body for use as an energy source during normal body system operation.

Weight Training

Women over 50 can also benefit from the improved bone health that comes from weight training. Weight lifting is significant for women over 50 years old as this is a time when your body begins to deteriorate. The weight lifting you do helps build and repair your muscles, which is an important part of having a healthy body in your fifties. It is also very important that you maintain a healthy diet while doing weight lifting, as an imbalanced diet can slow down the effectiveness of weight training or even result in negative side effects such as sore joints or muscles, headaches and other discomforts.

Weight lifting can be done several times per week for 30 minutes. If you are doing weight lifting and cardio exercise 2 to 3 times per week, it will be beneficial to do this in the morning to start your day off as this will get your metabolism going and improve your body's overall health. Women over 50 years old should have no problem losing weight due to weight lifting and working out.

You can also take advantage of free weights at home or visit a gym for a strength training class. A good strength training routine for women over 50 years old consists of 4 sets of 10 to 12 repetitions with 1-minute rest between each set.

Weight training will help you keep a healthy weight and improve your metabolism. You should do strength training 1 to 2 times per week for 30 minutes to 45 minutes.

Exercises That You Can Do at Home

For women who don't have the time to go to the gym, you can do a lot of exercises at home and still be able to lose weight.

Yoga

Yoga is a good one for women over 50 years old as it helps with flexibility. It can also help you in other ways, such as improving your sleep. If you need more energy throughout the day, try doing yoga during the morning hours instead of doing cardio exercise first thing in the morning. Some aerobic exercises can actually be counterproductive if they are done too soon after eating breakfast.

You can do yoga at home by following a DVD, and it can be done in the morning or evening. For women over 50, yoga is a good option that will help them lose weight and stay healthy.

Calisthenics

Calisthenics is ideal for women over 50 years old who want to lose weight fast. This refers to exercises such as push-ups, pull-ups, sit-ups and squats that can be done without any equipment. Calisthenics is very simple to do at home and can help you lose weight quite quickly. You can do calisthenics in the morning, evening or even at night before you go to bed.

Dance

Dancing can also be a good option for women over 50 years old who don't have a lot of time because it burns calories and is fun to do. Dancing does not only refer to ballroom dancing but any type of dance you might enjoy doing. It can help you with balance, flexibility and getting more exercise into your day. It is not necessary to be a professional to do so. You can just pick up a dance class at the community gym or borrow one of your friend's classes from time to time.

Aerobics

Aerobics refers to an aerobic exercise routine that involves rhythmic movements performed using our own body weight and muscle power to burn calories. The benefits of aerobics are improved posture, body tone, better cardiovascular health and increased flexibility and energy levels.

Chapter 12
Spirulina Algae: The Supplement That Helps Your Fast

When you want to lose weight and you do not want to have to consume a ton of calories and struggle with your diet, the best bet is to try Spirulina algae. This is due to the high protein and carbohydrate content, which will help your body feel fuller for a longer period of time. It also has been shown in many studies that it can help reduce or prevent the development of type 2 diabetes. This natural supplement can be taken either in powder form or through capsules, so there are no issues with trying different kinds of packaging. You can find this product at almost any vitamin or supplement store. It is also very affordable. You should be able to purchase large containers for $20-$30 apiece.

How Does It Work?

Spirulina algae, which is high in nutrients, helps your body feel full for a longer period of time, which means you won't have to consume as many calories when trying to lose weight.

In addition, it has been shown that this supplement is high in antioxidants and vitamin A, B-complex vitamins, and other essential nutrients like iron. This means that it will help boost your immune system and improve the health of your hair and nails as well. Spirulina also has been linked with the development of type 2 diabetes. Many studies have shown that those who eat a high amount of this supplement have a lower chance of developing and/or keeping the disease. This means that you can use it as an energy boost and get the added benefits of vitamins, minerals, and overall health benefits without worrying about it turning into a disease.

The Risks of Consuming Spirulina Algae

The main risk of using this product is that it can cause significant discomfort for some people. This happens when you take large amounts because you will feel bloated or gassy, which can make you want to throw up. In addition, in rare cases it can cause some people to experience skin rashes and/or have an allergic reaction, so make sure that you do not take it if you are allergic to any type of spirulina or seaweed. If your skin does get irritated after taking this supplement you should not use it for about two weeks and then start using very small amounts as a test before increasing the dosage.

Long-Term and Short-Term Advantages of Spirulina Algae

When taken over a long period of time, this supplement can help you lose weight while also improving your overall health and preventing disease. You will also feel better because as it can help your body digest food more efficiently and keep you fuller for longer, it will increase your energy levels. This is especially helpful if you're trying to lose weight but aren't getting enough calories. It can also help to improve your mood, which may be caused by increased energy levels during the day.

How to Use Spirulina Algae

When taking this supplement, it is very important that you use the recommended dose and ingredients listed on the bottle or container of Spirulina algae that you get. Do not assume that one bottle of this product contains the same amount of nutrients as other brands of Spirulina algae, so do not buy from anyone other than a reputable vitamin store or supplement shop. When you have it, you can take it as often as you want when you're trying to lose weight. You can also take several capsules of this product each day to increase your energy levels. When taking this supplement, make sure that you take it with a high-protein snack like nuts or protein bars that have a lot of protein so that you do not experience any discomfort from bloating.

Chapter 13. What to Avoid and What to Eat

What to Eat

Berries

Berries are very healthy, incredibly flavorful, and much lower in calories and sugar than you might think! Their tart sweetness can bring a smoothie to life, and they make a delicious snack on their own without any help from things like cream or sugar.

Cruciferous Vegetables

These are vegetables like cabbage, Brussels sprouts, broccoli, and cauliflower. These are beautiful additions to your diet because they're packed with vital nutrients and fiber that your body will love and use quickly!

Eggs

Eggs are such a great addition to your diet because they're packed to the gills with protein, you can do just about anything with them, they're easy to prepare, travel well if you hard boil them, and they can pair with just about anything. They're an excellent protein source for salads, and they're right on their own as well.

Fish

In particular, whitefish is typically very lean, but fish like salmon that have a little bit of color in them are packed with protein, fats, and oils that are great for you. They're good for brain and heart health, and there's a massive array of delicious things you can do with them.

Healthy Starches Like Individual Potatoes (With Skins!)

In particular, red potatoes are excellent to eat, even if you're trying to lose weight because your body can use those carbs for fuel, and the skins are packed with minerals that your body will enjoy. A little bit of potato here and there can do good things for your nutrition, but they are also a great way to feel like you're getting a little more of those fun foods that you should cut back on.

Legumes

Beans, the magical fruit. They're packed with protein, and the starch in them makes them stick to your ribs without making you pay for it later. They're lovely in soups, salads, and just about any other meal of the day that you're looking to fill out.

By adding beans to your regimen, you might find that your meals stick with you a little bit longer and leave you feeling more satisfied than you thought possible.

Nuts

I know you've heard people talking about how a handful of almonds makes a great snack, and if you're anything like me, you've always had kind of a hard time believing it. Nuts, as it turns out, have a good deal of their healthy fats in them that your body can use to get through those rough patches and, while they were not the most satisfying snack on their own, you might consider topping your salad with them for a little bit of crunch, or pairing them with some berries to make them a little more satisfying.

Probiotics Help Boost Your Gut Health

Having a happy gut often means that your dietary success and overall health will improve!

Vegetables That Are Rich in Healthy Fats

Not to sound topical or trendy, but avocados are a great example of a vegetable packed with healthy fats. Look for vegetables with fatty acids and a higher fat content and you will find that if you add more of those into your regimen, you will get hungry less often.

Water, Water, Water, and More Water

No matter what you decide to add to or subtract from your regimen, stay hydrated. It will help digestive health and ease, and it will keep you from feeling slump or tired, keeping you from getting too hungry. Add electrolytes where you need to, and don't be shy about bringing a bottle with you when you go from place to place. Stay hydrated!

What to Avoid

Grains

Whole grains may have their health benefits and be full of fiber, and you can also get these nutrients elsewhere. The human diet does not require grain consumption. The truth is while grains may have some benefits, they are ridiculously high in both total and net carbohydrates, making them incompatible with the ketogenic diet.

Some people do try what is known as the targeted ketogenic diet, which is a version of the diet specifically designed for those who complete extended and strenuous workouts. With the targeted ketogenic diet, a person will consume a small serving of carb-heavy food, such as grains, for 30 to 40 minutes before working out.

Starchy Vegetables and Legumes

Some vegetables are high in carbohydrates. It includes potatoes, beans, beets, corn, and more. These vegetables may have nutritional benefits, but you can get these same nutrients in low-carb vegetable alternatives.

Sugary Fruits

Most fruits contain a high sugar content, meaning that they are also high in carbohydrates. It is important to avoid most fruits. The exception is that you can enjoy berries, lemons, and limes in moderation. Some people will also enjoy a small serving of melon as a treat from time to time, but watch your portion size as it can add up quickly!

Milk and Low-Fat Dairy Products

As you can enjoy dairy products such as cheese on the ketogenic diet, you may consider trying milk. Sadly, milk is much higher in carbohydrates than cheese, with a glass of two-percent milk containing twelve carbs, half of your daily total. Instead, choose low-carb and dairy-free milk alternatives such as almond, coconut, and soy milk.

You may consider using low-fat cheeses instead of full fat to reduce the saturated fats you are consuming. The reason for this is that when the cheese is made with low-fat dairy, it naturally has a higher carbohydrate content, which will cut into your daily net carb total.

Cashews, Pistachios, and Chestnuts

While you can enjoy nuts and seeds in moderation, keep in mind that nuts contain a moderate carbohydrate level and therefore should be eaten in moderation. However, some nuts are high in carbs and thus are not fed on the ketogenic diet, including cashews, pistachios, and chestnuts. If you want to enjoy nuts, you can fully enjoy almonds, pecans, walnuts, macadamia nuts, and other options instead of these options.

Most Natural Sweeteners

While you can undoubtedly enjoy sugar-free natural sweeteners such as stevia, monk fruit, and sugar alcohols, you should avoid natural sweeteners that contain sugar. Suffice to say, and the sugar content makes these sweeteners naturally high in carbs. But not only that, but they will also spike your blood sugar and insulin. It means you should avoid things such as honey, agave, maple, coconut palm sugar, and dates.

Alcohol

Alcohol is not generally enjoyed on the ketogenic diet as your body will be unable to burn off calories while your liver attempts to process alcohol. Many people also find that when they are in ketosis, they get drunk more quickly and experience more severe hangovers. Not only that, but alcohol adds unnecessary calories and carbohydrates to your diet.

The worst offenders to choose would be margaritas, piña coladas, sangrias, Bloody Mary, whiskey sours, cosmopolitans, and regular beers. But, if you choose to drink alcohol regardless of drink in moderation and choose low-carb versions such as rum, vodka, tequila, whiskey, and gin. The next best options would be dry wines and light beers.

Chapter 14
Breakfast Recipes

1. Trail Mix

Preparation time: 5 minutes.

Cooking time: 0 minutes.

Servings: 6

Ingredients:

- 1 c. sunflower seeds (raw).
- 1 c. almonds (raw).
- 1 c. raisins.
- ¼ c. flaked coconut (optional).
- ½ c. dried apricot (unsulphured, chopped).
- ¼ c. carob chips (optional) or ¼ c. chocolate (optional).

Directions:

1. Pour it all into a big container, cover it and shake it!

2. Store in a bag that is airtight. To preserve the properties of the essential fatty acids, place them in the fridge/freezer.

Nutrition:

- **Calories:** 232 kcal.
- **Protein:** 6.18 g.
- **Fat:** 12.44 g.
- **Carbohydrates:** 27.97 g.

3. Warm Roasted Vegetable Farro Salad

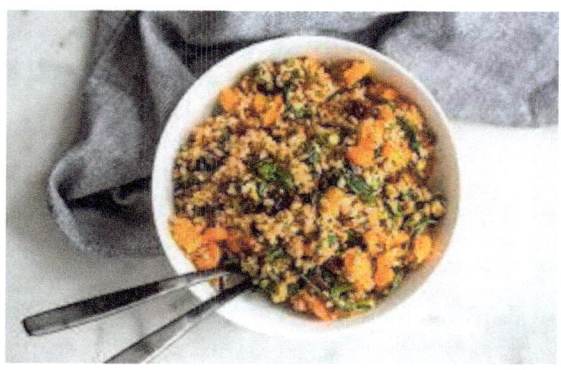

Preparation time: 30 minutes.

Cooking time: 1 hour and 5 minutes.

Servings: 4

Ingredients:

- 1 tbsp kosher salt or 1 tbsp sea salt.
- ½ medium-sized eggplant, peel on, and large diced.
- 1 c. cherry tomatoes washed and left whole.
- 6 white button mushrooms, quartered.
- 1 medium-sized zucchini, peel on, and large diced.
- 6 garlic cloves, peeled, trimmed, and sliced.

- ½ medium-sized red onion, peeled and cut into wedges.

- 1 c. cracked farro.

- 2 c. almond milk (Almond Breeze).

- 2 tbsp olive oil + 1 tsp olive oil.

- 1 tbsp balsamic vinegar.

- 3 sprigs fresh cilantro.

- ½ tsp salt.

- ½ tsp pepper.

Directions:

1. Preheat the oven to 400°F.

2. Salt the eggplant slices generously on all sides in a wide flat pan or baking sheet, toss to cover evenly, and keep for 30 minutes to release excess moisture and bitterness.

3. Drain the eggplant and rinse and toss it into a large mixing bowl. Tomatoes, zucchini, mushrooms, garlic, and onions are added. Drizzle the vegetables with olive oil generously, season with salt and pepper, and stir to coat. Move the vegetables to a pan lined with ovenproof tin foil. In the oven, roast the vegetables for 20 to 25 minutes or until tender, caramelized, and forked. To avoid sticking to the plate, stir or flip the vegetables about 10 to 15 minutes into the roasting

process. Set aside and remove the pan from the oven.

4. Meanwhile, rinse the farro with water and drain over the sink in a colander. Into a 3-quart (3L) saucepot, add the farro and add in the Almond Breeze. A pinch of salt and a drizzle of olive oil is added. Bring the liquid to a boil over medium-high heat to prevent boiling, then turn the heat down to a gentle simmer. Simmer the farro with the lid on the pot cocked to one side for 20 minutes to let out steam. Turn off the heat but leave the pot and close the lid on the stovetop. For another 5 minutes or until the farro is soft yet slightly chewy in the middle, steam in the pot. I was using a fork to loosen the lid and the fluff.

5. Mix the cooked farro with the vegetables in a large serving dish and gently toss to mix until ready to assemble the dish. Whisk the balsamic vinegar along with the olive oil and drizzle over the farro salad. Toss to coat and season to taste with salt and pepper. Add fresh cilantro and a squeeze of lemon to garnish. Serve it sweet.

Nutrition:

- **Calories:** 127 kcal.
- **Protein:** 2.17 g.
- **Fat:** 8.22 g.
- **Carbohydrates:** 13.29 g.

3. Cajun Potato, Prawn/Shrimp, and Avocado Salad

Preparation time: 10 minutes.

Cooking time: 20 minutes.

Servings: 2

Ingredients:

- 1 tbsp olive oil.
- 300 g. new potatoes (small baby or chats 10 oz. halved).
- 250 g. king prawns (8 oz., cooked and peeled).
- 2 spring onions (finely sliced).
- 1 garlic clove (minced).
- 2 tsps Cajun seasoning.
- 1 c. alfalfa sprout.
- 1 avocado (peeled, stoned, and diced).
- Salt (to boil potatoes).

Directions:

1. Cook the potatoes for 10 to 15 minutes in a large saucepan of lightly salted boiling water, or until tender, and then drain well.

2. In a wok or a large nonstick frying pan/skillet, heat the oil.

3. Season with the prawns, garlic, spring onions, and Cajun and fry for 2 to 3 minutes or until the prawns are hot.

4. Stir in the potatoes, and then cook for an additional minute.

5. Transfer to dishes for serving and top with the avocado and sprouts of alfalfa and eat.

Nutrition:

- **Calories:** 300 kcal.
- **Protein:** 19.08 g.
- **Fat:** 17.2 g.
- **Carbohydrates:** 18.51 g.

4. Baked Mahi-Mahi

Preparation time: 15 minutes.

Cooking time: 25 minutes.

Servings: 4

Ingredients:

- 2 lbs. mahi-mahi (4 fillets).
- ¼ tsp garlic salt.
- 1 lemon, juiced.
- 1 c. mayonnaise.
- ¼ c. white onion, finely chopped.
- ¼ tsp ground black pepper.
- 1 c. breadcrumbs.

Directions:

1. Preheat the oven to 425°F.

2. Put it in a baking dish and rinse the fish. Squeeze the fish with lemon juice and sprinkle with garlic salt and pepper.

3. Combine the mayonnaise and the chopped onions and scatter them over the fish. Sprinkle with breadcrumbs and bake for 25 minutes at 425°F.

Nutrition:

- **Calories:** 912 kcal.
- **Protein:** 56.77 g.
- **Fat:** 62.04 g.
- **Carbohydrates:** 32.48 g.

5. Sheet Pan Chicken and Brussel Sprouts

Preparation time: 5 minutes.

Cooking time: 35 minutes.

Servings: 4

Ingredients:

- 1 ½ c. Brussels sprouts, halved.
- 4 skin-on chicken thighs.
- 4 carrots, cut on the bias.
- 1 tsp herbs de Provence.
- 3 tbsp olive oil.
- ½ tsp salt.
- ½ tsp freshly ground black pepper.

Directions:

1. Preheat the stove to 400°F.

2. Put the cut vegetables in a bowl and add 1 ½ tbsps of olive oil, ½ tbsps of herbs, salt, and pepper. Rub the vegetables all over.

3. On a sheet pan, place the veggies.

4. In the same bowl, add the chicken thighs. Drizzle with 1 ½ tbsps of olive oil, ½ tbsps of herbs, salt, and pepper. Rub the chicken all over.

5. Put the chicken in a pan.

6. Roast for 30 to 35 minutes or until you are done with the chicken.

7. Turn the oven over to broil and cook for 1 to 2 minutes if you prefer a crispier vegetable or chicken skin. Carefully watch, or it will burn.

Nutrition:

- **Calories:** 152 kcal.
- **Protein:** 8.86 g.
- **Fat:** 11.49 g.
- **Carbohydrates:** 3.55 g.

6. Perfect Cauliflower Pizza Crust

Preparation time: 10 minutes.

Cooking time: 1 hour.

Servings: 4

Ingredients:

- 1 egg, beaten.
- 4 c. raw cauliflower, riced, or 1 medium cauliflower head.
- 1 c. goat cheese or 1 c. other soft cheese.
- 1 pinch of salt.
- 1 tsp dried oregano.

Directions:

1. Preheat to 400°F in your oven.
2. Pulse batches of raw cauliflower florets in a food processor to render the cauliflower rice until a rice-like texture is achieved.
3. Fill a big pot and bring it to a boil with around 1-inch of water. Add the "rice" and cover; cook for 5 minutes or so. Drain the strainer into a fine-mesh one.
4. **This is the secret:** Move it to a clean, thin dishtowel once you have strained the rice. In the

dishtowel, cover the steamed rice, curl it and suck out all the excess moisture! It is incredible how much extra liquid will be released, leaving you with an excellent dry crust of the pizza.

5. Mix your strained rice, beaten egg, goat's cheese, and spices in a big bowl. (Don't fear using your hands! You want it mixed well.) It is not going to be like every pizza dough you have ever dealt with, yet don't worry, it is going to stay together!

6. On a baking sheet lined with parchment paper, press the dough out. Keep the dough about $3/8$-inch thick, and make the edges a little higher for a "crust" effect, if you like. (It must be lined with parchment paper, or it will stick.)

7. Bake at 400°F for 35 to 40 minutes. The crust should be firm and, when done, golden brown.

8. Now's the time to add sauce, cheese, and any other toppings you want to all your favorites. Put the pizza back in the oven for 400°F and bake for an additional 5 to 10 minutes, only until the cheese is hot and bubbly.

9. Cut and quickly serve!

Nutrition:

- **Calories:** 76 kcal.
- **Protein:** 7.28 g.
- **Fat:** 2.71 g.
- **Carbohydrates:** 6.13 g.

8. Sweet Potato and Black Bean Burrito

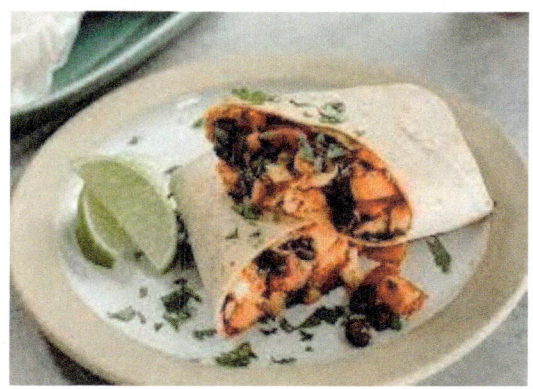

Preparation time: 10 minutes.

Cooking time: 1 hour.

Servings: 8 to 12

Ingredients:

- 5 c. peeled cubed sweet potatoes.
- 2 tsps other vegetable oil or 2 tsps broth.
- ½ tsp salt.
- 3 ½ c. diced onions.
- 1 tbsp minced fresh green chili pepper.

- 4 garlic cloves, minced (or pressed).
- 4 tsps ground cumin.
- 4 ½ c. cooked black beans (3 15 oz. cans, drained).
- 4 tsps ground coriander.
- ²⁄₃ c. lightly packed cilantro leaf.
- 1 tsp salt.
- 12 (10 inches) flour tortillas.
- 2 tbsp fresh lemon juice.
- Fresh salsa.

Directions:

1. Preheat the oven to 350°F.
2. Place the salt and water in a medium saucepan to cover the sweet potatoes.
3. Cover and bring to a boil, then simmer for about 10 minutes, until tender.
4. Drain yourself and set aside.
5. Heat the oil in a medium saucepan or skillet while the sweet potatoes are frying, and add the onions, garlic, and chili.
6. On medium-low heat, cover and cook, occasionally stirring, until the onions are tender, around 7 minutes.

7. Add cumin and coriander and cook, frequently stirring, for 2 to 3 minutes longer.

8. Remove and set aside from the sun.

9. Combine the black beans, lemon juice, cilantro, salt, and cooked sweet potatoes in a food processor and puree until smooth (or mash the ingredients in a large bowl by hand).

10. In a large mixing bowl, pass the sweet potato mixture and blend in the cooked onions and spices.

11. Oil a large baking dish lightly.

12. At the center of each tortilla, spoon around $2/3$ to $3/4$ c. of the filling, roll it up, and put it in the baking dish, seam side down.

13. Cover thoroughly with foil and bake for 30 minutes or so, until sweet.

14. Serve with salsa topping.

Nutrition:

- **Calories:** 208 kcal.
- **Protein:** 6.76 g.
- **Fat:** 4.1 g.
- **Carbohydrates:** 36.42 g.

8. Crockpot Black-Eyed Peas

Preparation time: 5 minutes.

Cooking time: 10 hours.

Servings: 6

Ingredients:

- 1 small ham hock.
- 1 (16 oz.) bag dried black-eyed peas.
- 1 (14 ½ oz.) can have diced tomatoes with green chilies.
- 1 (14 ½ oz.) can Del Monte diced tomato with zesty jalapeno and pepper.
- 1 stalk celery, chopped.
- 2 (10 ½ oz.) can of chicken broth.

Directions:

1. Following the directions on the bag, pre-soak black-eyed peas.
2. Combine all ingredients and cook for 9 to 10 hours on low heat.

Nutrition:

- **Calories:** 145 kcal.
- **Protein:** 22.24 g.
- **Fat:** 5.3 g.
- **Carbohydrates:** 1.81 g.

9. Peach Berry Smoothie

Preparation time: 5 minutes.

Cooking time: 0 minutes.

Servings: 1

Ingredients:

- 1 c. frozen peaches.
- ¼ c. coconut milk (adjust for a thicker or thinner smoothie).
- ½ tsp almond flavoring.
- 2 oz. Greek yogurt.

Directions:

1. In a high-speed blender, blend the peaches, Greek yogurt with almond flavoring.
2. Check and change the thickness accordingly. For thinner, add more milk, and for thicker, more peaches.
3. Gorgeous toppings such as chia seeds, berries, and slivered almonds are on top. Enjoy.

Nutrition:

- **Calories:** 478 kcal.
- **Protein:** 6.54 g.
- **Fat:** 36.6 g.
- **Carbohydrates:** 39.12 g.

10. Sweet Potato Curry with Spinach and Chickpeas

Preparation time: 5 minutes.

Cooking time: 25 minutes.

Servings: 6

Ingredients:

- 1 to 2 tsps canola oil.
- 1 tbsp cumin.
- 2 tbsp curry powder.
- 1 tsp cinnamon.
- ½ large sweet onions, chopped, or 2 scallions, thinly sliced.
- 10 oz. fresh spinach washed, stemmed, and coarsely chopped.
- 1 (14 ½ oz.) can chickpeas, rinsed and drained.
- 2 large sweet potatoes, peeled and diced (about 2 lbs.)
- ½ c. water.
- ¼ c. chopped fresh cilantro for garnish.
- 1 (14 ½ oz.) can diced tomatoes, can substitute fresh if available.

- Basmati rice or brown rice, for serving.

Directions:

1. Whatever you like, you can choose to cook sweet potatoes. I enjoy peeling, slicing, and steaming mine for about 15 minutes in a veggie steamer. Fit well baking or boiling, too.

2. Heat 1 to 2 tsps of canola or vegetable oil over medium heat while the sweet potatoes are cooking.

3. Add the onions and sauté for 2 to 3 minutes, or until tender.

4. Add the curry powder, cumin, and cinnamon, and then stir to cover the spices' onions evenly.

5. Stir in the tomatoes and their juices, and stir in the chickpeas to blend.

6. Add ½ c. of water and lift the heat for about 1 to 2 minutes to a high simmer.

7. Then add fresh spinach, stirring to cover with cooking liquid, a few handfuls at a time.

8. Cover and boil until just wilted, about 3 minutes, when all the spinach is added to the pan.

9. Apply to the liquid the cooked sweet potatoes, and stir to coat.

10. Simmer for another 3 to 5 minutes, or until you mix the flavors nicely.

11. Move to a dish for serving, toss with fresh cilantro and serve sweet.

12. This dish is served beautifully over basmati or brown rice.

Nutrition:

- **Calories:** 111 kcal.
- **Protein:** 4.36 g.
- **Fat:** 2.83 g.
- **Carbohydrates:** 18.46 g.

11. Poached Eggs and Avocado Toasts

Preparation time: 15 minutes.

Cooking time: 0 minutes.

Servings: 4

Ingredients:

- 2 ripe avocados.
- 4 eggs.
- 2 tsps lemon juice (or juice of 1 lime).
- 1 c. cheese (grated, edam, gruyere, or whatever you have on hand).
- 4 slices of thick bread.
- 4 tsps butter (for spreading on toast).
- Salt and freshly ground black pepper.

Directions:

1. Using your favorite technique, poach eggs.
2. Meanwhile, the avocados are cut in half, and the stones are removed.
3. Scoop out the flesh in a bowl with a spoon and apply the lemon or lime juice, salt, and pepper.
4. Mash using a fork.

5. Bread toast and spread with butter.

6. On each slice of buttered toast, spread the avocado mix and top each one with 1 poached egg.

7. Sprinkle the grated cheese over it and serve immediately.

8. These are also good with tomato halves on the side, either fresh or grilled.

Nutrition:

- **Calories:** 258 kcal.
- **Protein:** 11.78 g.
- **Fat:** 20.89 g.
- **Carbohydrates:** 7.32 g.

12. Sweet Potato Hash

Preparation time: 10 minutes.

Cooking time: 30 minutes.

Servings: 4

Ingredients:

- ½ tsp cumin.
- ½ tsp salt.
- 1 lg. bell pepper, diced.
- 1 med. onion, diced.
- 1 tsp garlic powder.
- 1.5 lb. sweet potatoes, cubed.
- 2 c. frozen spinach, chopped, thawed, & drained.
- 2 med. green onions, sliced.
- 2 tbsp avocado oil (or oil of preference).
- 4 lg. eggs.
- 6 oz. turkey sausage, halved & sliced.
- Ground black pepper, to taste.
- Red pepper flakes, to taste.

Directions:

1. Heat a large skillet over medium-high heat and warm the oil in the pan, spreading it evenly over the bottom of the pan.

2. Stir the onion and bell peppers into the pan and heat through until shiny and fragrant, about 3 minutes.

3. Stir the sausage into the pan along with the garlic powder, sweet potatoes, cumin, pepper flakes, ground pepper, and salt.

4. Stir all ingredients to fully incorporate, then cover the skillet and allow to cook on low heat for 12 to 15 minutes, stirring a few times throughout. The potatoes should be firm, but cooked.

5. Stir the spinach into the pan until completely incorporated.

6. Using your spoon or spatula, make 4 little divots or wells into the mixture and crack 1 egg into each well. Season to taste then cover and allow to cook for another 5 minutes or so until the eggs have reached the desired level of doneness.

7. Garnish with green onion and serve hot!

Nutrition:

- **Calories:** 390 kcal.
- **Protein:** 17 g.
- **Fat:** 16 g.
- **Carbohydrates:** 44 g.
- **Sugar:** 14 g.

13. Blueberry Smoothie

Preparation time: 5 minutes.

Cooking time: 0 minutes.

Servings: 1

Ingredients:

- ½ c. quick oats.
- 1 ½ c. almond milk, unsweetened.
- 1 c. blueberries, fresh or frozen.
- 1 scoop nutritional shake powder.

Directions:

1. Combine all ingredients into a blender and blend until completely smooth, scraping down the sides of the jar as needed.
2. Serve cold!

Nutrition:

- **Calories:** 442 kcal.
- **Protein:** 29 g.
- **Fat:** 13 g.
- **Carbohydrates:** 62 g.
- **Sugar:** 16 g.

14. Almond Smoothie

Preparation time: 5 minutes.

Cooking time: 0 minutes.

Servings: 1

Ingredients:

- ¼ c. almonds, raw & unsalted.
- ½ c. quick oats.
- ½ tsp almond extract.
- 1 ¼ c. almond milk, unsweetened.
- 2 scoops vanilla protein powder.

Directions:

1. Combine all ingredients into a blender and blend until completely smooth, scraping down the sides of the jar as needed.
2. Serve chilled!

Nutrition:

- **Calories:** 453 kcal.
- **Protein:** 31 g.
- **Fat:** 24 g.
- **Carbohydrates:** 30 g.
- **Sugar:** 4 g.

Chapter 15. Lunch Recipes

15. Herb-Roasted Chicken Breasts

Preparation time: 4 hours.

Cooking time: 20 minutes.

Servings: 4

Ingredients:

- 1 onion.
- 4 c. of chicken breasts (boneless and skinless).
- 1 to 2 cloves of garlic.
- 1 tsp ground black pepper.
- ¼ c. olive oil.
- 2 tbsp garlic & herb seasoning (no salt added).

Directions:

1. In a bowl, chop garlic, onion, add herb seasoning, olive oil, and pepper.
2. Add chicken to this mix, cover with plastic wrap, then chill in the fridge for 4 hours.
3. Let the oven preheat to 350°F.

4. Place marinated chicken on foil on a baking tray

5. Add the marinade over chicken and bake for 20 minutes

For browning:

1. Broil for 5 minutes.

Nutrition:

- **Calories:** 270 kcal.
- **Protein:** 26 g.
- **Total fat:** 17 g.
- **Carbohydrates:** 3 g.
- **Cholesterol:** 83 mg.
- **Sodium:** 53 mg.
- **Phosphorus:** 252 mg.
- **Dietary fiber:** 0.6 g.

16. Zesty Chicken

Preparation time: 30 minutes to 24 hours.

Cooking time: 30 to 40 minutes.

Servings: 2

Ingredients:

- 2 tbsp olive oil.
- 2 tbsp balsamic vinegar.
- ¼ c. green onion.
- ¼ tsp paprika.
- 8 oz. chicken breast (skinless and boneless).
- ¼ tsp black pepper.
- 1 tsp fresh oregano.
- ½ tsp garlic powder.

Directions:

1. In a mug, whisk olive oil and balsamic vinegar. Add chopped green onion, herbs, and seasoning, mix well. Cut chicken into 2 pieces.

2. In a zip lock bag, add chicken and pour marinade over. Let it chill in the fridge for 30 minutes to 24 hours.

3. Grease the pan, cook chicken until chicken's internal temperature reaches 170°F

Nutrition:

- **Calories:** 280 kcal.
- **Protein:** 27 g.
- **Fat:** 16 g.
- **Carbohydrates:** 4 g.
- **Cholesterol:** 73 mg.
- **Sodium:** 68 mg.
- **Calcium:** 26 mg.
- **Fiber:** 0.3 g.

17. Chicken Quinoa Anti-Inflammatory

Preparation time: 25 minutes.

Cooking time: 14 to 18 minutes.

Servings: 4

Ingredients:

- 4 tbsp olive oil divided.
- 1-pound boneless, skinless chicken breasts.
- ¼ c. finely chopped red onion.
- 2 c. roasted red peppers.
- 1 minced garlic clove.
- 1 tsp paprika.
- ¼ tsp crushed red pepper (optional).
- 2 c. cooked quinoa.
- ½ tsp ground cumin.
- ¼ c. olives, chopped.
- 1 c. diced cucumber.
- 1 c. diced tomato
- ¼ c. almonds.
- ¼ c. crumbled feta cheese.

- ¼ tsp salt.
- ¼ tsp ground pepper.
- 2 tbsp fresh parsley.

Directions:

1. In the upper third of the oven, put a rack; let the broiler preheat. Place foil on a rimmed baking dish.
2. Put salt and pepper on the chicken, and put it on the prepared baking sheet. Broil it for 14 to 18 min, rotating once, till a thermometer instant-read added in the thickest section registers 165°F. Move the chicken and slice on a cutting board.
3. Meanwhile, put 2 spoons of oil, cumin, peppers, almonds, crushed red pepper and paprika in a food processor. Pulse it until creamy
4. In a medium dish, mix olives, quinoa, 2 spoons of oil, and red onion. mix it well
5. Divide the quinoa mixture into 4 bowls and finish with similar quantities of red pepper sauce, cucumber, and tomato to eat. Sprinkle with parsley and feta.
6. Enjoy.

Nutrition:

- **Calories:** 219 kcal.
- **Protein:** 34.1 g.
- **Total fat:** 26.9 g.
- **Carbohydrates:** 31.2 g.
- **Potassium:** 187 mg.
- **Phosphorus:** 132 mg.

18. Skillet Lemon Chicken & Potatoes with Kale

Preparation time: 20 minutes.

Cooking time: 25 minutes.

Servings: 4

Ingredients:

- 1 tbsp chopped tarragon.
- 1-pound boneless, skinless chicken thighs (trimmed).
- ½ tsp ground pepper (divided)
- 3 tbsp olive oil.
- ½ tsp salt (divided).
- ½ c. light chicken broth.
- 6 c. baby kale.
- 1 lemon (sliced).
- 4 cloves of garlic (minced).
- 1 pound baby Yukon gold potatoes; halved lengthwise (leached).

Directions:

1. Let the oven pre-heat till 400°F.

2. In a large skillet, heat 1 tbsp of oil.

3. Sprinkle with ¼ tsp of salt and pepper on chicken. Cook, rotating once, before browning on both sides, a total of about 5 minutes. Move into a tray.

4. Add ¼ tsp of salt and pepper to the pan with the remaining 2 tsps of oil, with potatoes.

5. Cook potatoes, cut-side down, for around 3 minutes, until browned. Add lemon, broth, garlic, and tarragon. Bring the chicken back into the pan.

6. Switch the frying pan to the oven.

7. Roast, about 15 minutes, before the chicken is completely cooked and the potatoes are soft.

8. Stir the kale into the mixture and roast for 3 to 4 minutes until it has wilted.

Nutrition:

- **Calories:** 347 kcal.
- **Protein:** 24.7 g.
- **Total fat:** 19.3 g.
- **Carbohydrates:** 25.6 g.
- **Potassium:** 171 mg.
- **Phosphorus:** 151 mg.

19. Grilled Chicken Salad with Mango & Avocado

Preparation time: 15 minutes.

Cooking time: 25 minutes.

Servings: 4

Ingredients:

- 1 ½ c. chicken breast (grilled and sliced).
- 2 tbsp red onion (diced).
- 1 c. diced mango.
- 6 c. baby lettuce, red butter.
- 1 c. diced avocado.

Vinaigrette:

- 2 tbsp white balsamic vinegar:
- 2 tbsp olive oil.
- ½ tsp turmeric.
- ¾ tsps fresh ginger.

Directions:

1. In a bowl, add all ingredients of vinaigrette, whisk well and set it aside.

2. In another bowl, add chicken, mango, onion, and avocado. Toss together.

3. In a serving platter, add baby greens on the bottom, add tossed salad on top, and drizzle with vinaigrette.

4. Toss and serve right away.

Nutrition:

One bowl:

- **Calories:** 321 kcals.
- **Protein:** 28.4 g.
- **Fat:** 7.1 g.
- **Carbohydrates:** 31 g.
- **Sodium:** 154 mg.
- **Cholesterol:** 28 mg.

20. Chicken & Snap Peas Stir Fry

Preparation time: 20 minutes.

Cooking time: 10 minutes.

Servings: 2 to 3

Ingredients:

- 1 ¼ c. skinless chicken breast (sliced).
- 2 tbsp vegetable oil.
- 2 minced garlic cloves.
- 2 ½ c. snap peas.
- Black pepper and salt
- 3 tbsp cilantro for garnish.
- 1 bunch of scallions (thinly sliced)
- 3 tbsp low sodium soy sauce.
- 1 red bell pepper(sliced)
- 2 tsps sriracha.
- 2 tsps. coriander
- 2 tbsp sesame seeds.
- 2 tbsp rice vinegar.

Directions:

1. Heat the oil over medium flame in a large pan. Stir in the garlic and scallions, then sauté for around 1 minute until fragrant. Stir in the snap peas and bell pepper, then sauté for 2 to 3 minutes until soft.

2. Add the chicken and cook for 4 to 5 minutes until golden and thoroughly cooked, and the vegetables are tender.

3. Add the sesame seeds, soy sauce, rice vinegar, sriracha, and mix well to blend. Allow boiling the mixture for 2 minutes.

4. Add the cilantro and garnish with coriander and sesame seeds. Serve hot

Nutrition:

- **Calories:** 228 kcal.
- **Protein:** 20 g.
- **Fat:** 11 g.
- **Carbohydrates:** 11 g.
- **Potassium:** 210 mg.
- **Phosphorus:** 105 mg.

21. Chicken Caprese Sandwich

Preparation time: 20 minutes.

Cooking time: 15 minutes.

Servings: 2 to 3

Ingredients:

- 4 tbsp, or more, extra virgin olive oil, divided.
- ½ lemon juiced.
- ¼ c. sliced fresh basil leaves.
- Kosher salt and freshly ground black pepper.
- 1 (8 oz.) log fresh mozzarella cheese, sliced into rounds (¼ thickness)
- 2 pieces of boneless chicken breasts (skinless)
- 1 tsp fresh parsley (sliced).
- 1 loaf (10 oz.) sourdough bread, cut in half lengthwise.
- Balsamic glaze or balsamic vinegar, to taste

Directions:

1. In a big mixing bowl, add parsley, black pepper, 2 tbsp of extra virgin olive oil, salt, lemon juice, mix it well. Pour this over chicken breasts and toss

lightly to coat well, and let the chicken rest at room temperature.

2. Put a grilling pan over medium heat. Add the chicken breast to the grilling pan, without the marinade, and add black pepper and salt. Flip the chicken after 4 minutes.

3. Cook for 3 minutes more, till grill marks appear.

4. Lower the flame, and cover the chicken and cook till the instant-read thermometer reads 185°F.

5. Turn off the heat and slice the chicken, and set it aside.

6. Pour 1 tbsp of extra-virgin olive oil into each side of the bread and grill it until golden brown.

7. Slice the bread into 3 slices for each half. Add 3 to 4 slices of chicken, few slices of mozzarella cheese to each slice. Pour balsamic vinegar, extra virgin olive oil on top. Add basil leaves on top.

8. Season with more salt and black pepper. Serve hot

Nutrition:

- **Calories:** 321 kcal.
- **Protein:** 34.42 g.
- **Fat:** 32.06 g.
- **Carbohydrates:** 46.88 g.
- **Potassium:** 210 mg.
- **Phosphorus:** 125 mg.

22. Zucchini Noodles with Pesto & Chicken

Preparation time: 15 minutes.

Cooking time: 10 minutes.

Servings: 4

Ingredients:

- 4 c. chicken breast, cut into bite-size pieces (boneless, skinless).
- ¼ c. extra-virgin olive oil and 2 tbsp more.
- 4 pieces of trimmed medium-large zucchini.
- ¼ c. shredded Parmesan cheese.
- 2 c. fresh basil (packed) leaves.
- 2 tbsp lemon juice.
- 1 large clove of chopped garlic.
- ¼ c. toasted pine nuts.
- ½ tsp freshly ground black pepper.
- ¾ tsp kosher salt, divided.

Directions:

1. Cut the zucchini in length into big, thin strands, utilizing a spiral vegetable slicer. Chops these long

noodles so the strands would not be very long. Put the zucchini in a colander, and add ¼ tsp of salt. Let it drain for almost 30 minutes, then press gently to extract any remaining moisture.

2. In a food processor bowl, add Parmesan, basil, ¼ tsp of salt, pine nuts, ¼ c. of olive oil, black pepper, lemon juice, and garlic, and pulse on high until smooth

3. Put a wide skillet over medium flame, add 1 tbsp of oil. Add chicken in an even layer, then add ¼ tsp of salt.

4. Let it cook, often stirring, for about 5 minutes. Then transfer to a bowl and stir in 3 tbsp of the pesto.

5. To the pan, add the remaining 1 tbsp of olive oil. Then add the dried zucchini noodles mix carefully for 2 to 3 minutes.

6. Add these noodles to the bowl with the cooked chicken. Add the leftover pesto and toss lightly to coat.

Nutrition:
- **Calories:** 430 kcal.
- **Protein:** 28.6 g
- **Total fat:** 31.6 g.
- **Carbohydrates:** 9.4 g.
- **Fiber:** 2.5 g.
- **Potassium:** 187 mg.
- **Phosphorus:** 143 mg.

23. Lettuce Wraps

Preparation time: 10 minutes.

Cooking time: 10 minutes.

Servings: 3 to 4

Ingredients:

For lettuce wraps:

- 3.6 c. minced turkey:
- 1 tbsp olive oil.
- 2 tsps dried minced onion.
- ¼ tsp sea salt.
- ¼ tsp black pepper.
- 3 green onions, thinly sliced.
- ¼ c. chopped shiitake mushrooms.
- ½ c. of diced jicama.
- Living butter lettuce.

For sauce:

- 3 tbsp soy sauce (less sodium).
- 2 cloves of garlic should be minced.
- ½ tsp ginger paste.

- 1 tsp sesame oil.
- 1 tsp rice vinegar.
- 1 tsp brown Swerve sweetener.
- 1 tsp almond butter, natural.

Directions:

1. Put all ingredients in a small bowl, whisk, and set aside.
2. Heat olive oil in a skillet on the stove. Crumble and cook the minced turkey on medium heat.
3. Season with chopped onion, sea salt, and black pepper.
4. Then add green onion, jicama, and mushrooms.
5. Add mushroom with meat until mushroom becomes soft—mix sauce with meat mixture.
6. Serve.

Nutrition:

- **Calories:** 188 kcal.
- **Proteins:** 26 g.
- **Fat:** 12 g.
- **Carbohydrates:** 9.4 g.
- **Fiber:** 5 g.
- **Potassium:** 157 mg.

24. Grilled Chicken Breast

Preparation time: 30 minutes.

Cooking time: 12 minutes.

Servings: 2

Ingredients:

- 4 pieces chicken breasts.

For the margination:

- 3 tsps olive oil.
- ¼ c. cilantro chopped.
- 2 cloves garlic minced.
- 1 lime juice.
- ½ tsp cumin.
- ½ tsp sea salt.
- ½ tsp paprika.
- ¼ tsp black pepper.

For avocado salsa:

- 2 small chopped tomatoes.
- ¼ c. chopped red onion.
- 1 jalapeno.

- ¼ c. cilantro, finely chopped.
- 2 diced avocados.
- 1 lime, juiced.
- Sea salt and black peppers.

Directions:

1. In a bowl, add all ingredients of marinade. Mix well and set it aside.
2. With a meat mallet, pound the chicken breast, and add to the marinade. Coat the chicken well in the marinade. Keep in the fridge for 30 minutes or overnight if you have time.
3. Preheat the grill pan over medium flame. Cook chicken for 5 to 6 minutes on each side or until cooked through and looks crispy on the outside.
4. Serve right away with avocado and fresh salsa and enjoy.

Salsa avocado:

1. In a bowl, add all ingredients of salsa. Meanwhile, the chicken is cooking. With plastic wrap, cover it and keep it in the fridge till serving time.
2. It is one of the delicious and easiest recipes to make.

Nutrition:

- **Calories:** 468 kcal.
- **Proteins:** 20 g.
- **Fat:** 10 g.
- **Carbohydrates:** 9.4 g.
- **Fiber:** 2 g.
- **Total fat:** 31.6 g.
- **Potassium:** 187 mg.
- **Sodium:** 91 mg.

25. Cheesy Chicken Salad

Preparation time: 35 minutes.

Cooking time: 0 minutes.

Servings: 1 to 2

Ingredients:

- 1 c., cooked chicken breast (skinless, boneless, cut into cubes)
- 2 ½ tbsps mayonnaise, fat-free.
- ¼ c. finely chopped celery.
- ½ c. fresh baby spinach, coarsely chopped.
- 2 tbsp sour cream (non-fat).
- ¼ c. carrot (shaved to ribbons).
- 2 tsps Dijon mustard.
- ¼ c. reduced-fat sharp cheddar cheese (shredded).
- ⅛ tsp dried parsley.

Directions:

1. In a mixing bowl, add all ingredients. Mix all ingredients well with a mayonnaise mixture.

2. Keep in the fridge for half an hour, or overnight if you prefer.

3. Serve and enjoy.

Nutrition:

- **Calories:** 364.5 kcal.
- **Protein:** 53.2 g.
- **Total fat:** 9.1 g.
- **Total carbohydrates:** 15.3 g.
- **Cholesterol:** 131.8 mg.
- **Dietary fiber:** 2.8 g.
- **Sugars:** 7.3 g.
- **Sodium:** 767.4 mg.

26. Chicken Breasts with Avocado Tapenade

Preparation time: 10 minutes.

Cooking time: 10 minutes.

Servings: 4

Ingredients:

- 5 tbsp fresh lemon juice, divided.
- 3 tbsp extra virgin olive oil, divided.
- 2 cloves of garlic, roasted and then mashed.
- 1 clove of finely chopped garlic.
- 1 tbsp freshly grated lemon peel.
- ¼ tsp salt.
- 4 skinless, boneless chicken breast cut in halves.
- ½ tsp fresh ground black pepper.
- 1 tomato, medium-sized, remove seeds, finely diced.
- 1 ripe avocado, large-sized, finely diced.
- 3 tbsp capers, rinsed.
- 2 tbsp fresh basil leaves, cut into fine slices.

- ¼ c. small-sized green pimento olive stuffed, cut into thin slices.

Directions:

1. In a zip lock bag, add 2 tbsp of lemon juice, garlic, black pepper, 2 tbsp of olive oil, ¼ tsp of salt, lemon peel, and chicken. Mix well and keep in the fridge for 30 minutes.

2. In a bowl, add roasted garlic, ¼ tsp of salt, ½ tsp of olive oil, 3 tbsp of lemon juice, black pepper. Mix and add in basil, green sliced olives, avocado, tomato, capers. Set it aside.

3. Take out the chicken from the bag, discard the marinade.

4. Preheat the grill on medium flame and cook chicken for 4 to 5 minutes on each side or until cooked through.

5. Serve grilled chicken with avocado salad.

Nutrition: 1 out of 4 servings:

- **Calories:** 277.1 kcal.
- **Protein:** 26.4 g.
- **Total fat:** 16.4 g.
- **Total carbohydrates:** 6.9 g.
- **Cholesterol:** 75.5 mg.
- **Sodium:** 914.6 mg.
- **Dietary fiber:** 3.1 g.

27. Beef & Barley Soup

Preparation time: 10 minutes.

Cooking time: 50 minutes.

Servings: 8

Ingredients:

- ½ c. parsley, finely chopped.
- ½ tsp thyme, dried.
- 1 c. wheat barley, hulled.
- 1 lb. ground beef.
- 1 lg. onion, diced.
- 1 tbsp extra virgin olive oil.
- 1 tsp salt.
- 2 lg. stalks celery, diced.
- 3 bay leaves.
- 3 cloves garlic, minced.
- 3 lg. carrots, diced.
- 9 c. low-sodium beef broth.
- Ground black pepper, to taste.

Directions:

1. Heat a large pot or Dutch oven over medium heat and add oil to it.

2. Once the oil is hot, stir the onion and garlic in, allowing them to cook for about 3 minutes, stirring often. Add barley.

3. Stir carrots, beef, celery, and thyme into the pot. Brown the beef, breaking it into smaller chunks as you do so.

4. Once the beef is browned, add the broth, salt, pepper, and bay leaves to the pot, stirring completely. Cover the pot and bring it to a boil.

5. Once boiling, reduce the heat to low and let simmer for 40 minutes.

6. Remove the pot from the heat and stir, adding the parsley and adjusting the seasoning to suit your taste. Remove the bay leaves and stir once more. Serve hot!

Nutrition:

- **Calories:** 189 kcal.
- **Protein:** 16 g.
- **Fat:** 4 g.
- **Carbohydrates:** 22 g.
- **Sugar:** 3 g.

28. Instant Pot Chicken

Preparation time: 5 minutes.

Cooking time: 20 minutes.

Servings: 6

Ingredients:

- 1 c. water.
- 1 tsp rosemary, chopped.
- 1 med. lemon, sliced.
- 2 cloves garlic, minced.
- 2 lb. chicken thighs, boneless & skinless.
- 2 tbsp extra virgin olive oil.
- Sea salt & pepper, to taste.

Directions:

1. Combine all ingredients in a medium mixing bowl, incorporate fully and cover.

2. Plug in your Instant Pot and select the Sauté setting. Drizzle a little extra olive oil into the bottom of it to prevent sticking.

3. Once the pot is hot, place the thighs in one even layer on the bottom of the Instant Pot and allow to cook until a golden crust is formed on the chick

(about 4 to 5 minutes), then flip and allow the other side to cook as well.

4. Pull the thighs out of the pot and use the water to deglaze the bottom of the pot, scraping lightly with your spatula or spoon as you stir the water around the pot.

5. Place the chicken into the pot (on top of the trivet insert if you have one, but no problem if you don't) and place the lid on top. Cook at high pressure for 5 minutes to cook the chicken the rest of the way through.

6. Release the pressure and remove the chicken from the pot.

7. Serve hot with your favorite sides!

Nutrition:

- **Calories:** 223 kcal.
- **Protein:** 30 g.
- **Fat:** 11 g.
- **Carbohydrates:** 0 g.
- **Sugar:** 0 g.

Chapter 16. Snack Recipes

29. Squash Bites

Preparation time: 10 minutes.

Cooking time: 40 minutes.

Servings: 4

Ingredients:

- 10 oz. turkey meat, cooked, sliced.
- 2 pounds of butternut squash, cubed.
- 1 tsp chili powder.
- 1 tsp garlic powder.
- 1 tsp sweet paprika.
- Black pepper to taste.

Directions:

1. In a bowl, mix butternut squash cubes with chili powder, black pepper, garlic powder, and paprika and toss to coat.

2. Wrap squash pieces in turkey slices, place them all on a lined baking sheet, place in the oven at 350°F, bake for 20 minutes, flip and bake for 20 minutes more.

3. Arrange squash bites on a platter and serve. Enjoy!

Nutrition:

- **Calories:** 223 kcal.
- **Protein:** 23 g.
- **Fat:** 3.8 g.
- **Carbohydrates:** 26.5 g.
- **Fiber:** 4.5 g.

30. Zucchini Chips

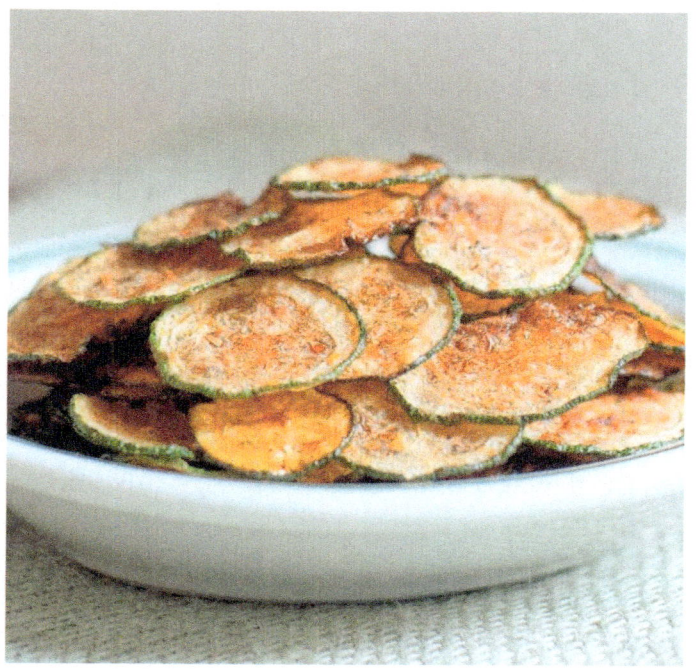

Preparation time: 10 minutes.

Cooking time: 12 minutes.

Servings: 4

Ingredients:

- 1 zucchini, thinly sliced.
- A pinch of sea salt.
- Black pepper, to taste.
- 1 tsp thyme, dried.

- 1 egg.
- 1 tsp garlic powder.
- 1 c. almond flour.

Directions:

1. In a bowl, whisk the egg with a pinch of salt.
2. Put the flour in another bowl and mix it with thyme, black pepper, and garlic powder.
3. Dredge zucchini slices in the egg mix and then in flour.
4. Arrange chips on a lined baking sheet, place in the oven at 450°F and bake for 6 minutes on each side,
5. Serve the zucchini chips as a snack. Enjoy!

Nutrition:

- **Calories:** 106 kcal.
- **Protein:** 5.1 g.
- **Fat:** 8.2 g.
- **Carbohydrates:** 5.2 g.
- **Fiber:** 2.1 g.

31. Pepperoni Bites

Preparation time: 5 minutes.

Cooking time: 10 minutes.

Servings: 24 pieces

Ingredients:

- 1/3 c. tomatoes, chopped.
- ½ c. bell peppers, mixed and chopped.
- 24 pepperoni slices.
- ½ c. tomato sauce.
- 4 oz. of almond cheese, cubed.
- 2 tbsp basil, chopped.
- Black pepper to taste.

Directions:

1. Divide pepperoni slices into a muffin tray.
2. Divide tomato and bell pepper pieces into the pepperoni cups.
3. Also divide the tomato sauce, basil and almond cheese cubes, sprinkle black pepper at the end, place cups in the oven at 400°F, and bake for 10 minutes.

4. Arrange the pepperoni bites on a platter and serve. Enjoy!

Nutrition:

- **Calories:** 59 kcal.

- **Protein:** 2.5 g.

- **Fat:** 4.5 g.

- **Carbohydrates:** 2 g.

- **Fiber:** 0.1 g.

32. Party Meatballs

Preparation time: 10 minutes.

Cooking time: 40 minutes.

Servings: 20

Ingredients:

- 1 pound of turkey meat, ground.
- 1 tbsp coconut oil, melted.
- 1 yellow onion, chopped.
- 1 egg.
- 1 c. of coconut flour.
- 1 tsp Italian seasoning.
- 1 tbsp hot sauce
- A pinch of sea salt.
- Black pepper to taste.
- 2 tbsp parsley, chopped.

Directions:

1. In a bowl, mix turkey meat with half of the flour, a pinch of salt, black pepper, Italian seasoning, parsley, onion, egg, and hot sauce and stir well.
2. Put the rest of the flour in another bowl.

3. Shape 20 turkey meatballs and dip each one in flour.

4. Heat up a pan with the oil over medium-high heat, add meatballs, cook them for 4 minutes on each side, transfer to paper towels to remove any excess grease, place all of them on a platter and serve. Enjoy!

Nutrition:

- **Calories:** 71 kcal.
- **Protein:** 7.7 g.
- **Fat:** 2.6 g.
- **Carbohydrates:** 4.1 g.
- **Fiber:** 2.2 g.

33. Chicken Strips

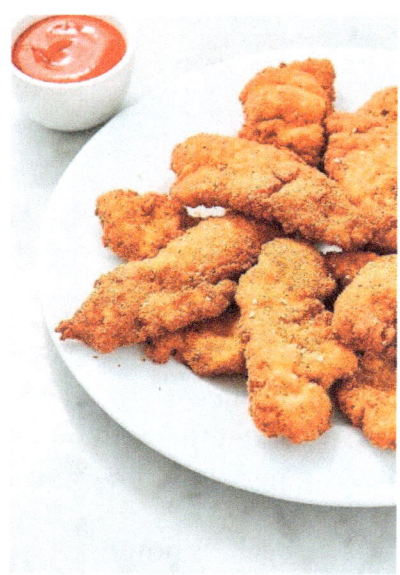

Preparation time: 10 minutes.

Cooking time: 20 minutes.

Servings: 4

Ingredients:

- 1-pound chicken tenders.
- 1 egg, whisked.
- A pinch of sea salt.
- $1/3$ c. coconut, unsweetened and shredded.

- ¼ c. coconut flour.

Directions:

1. In a bowl, mix coconut with coconut flour and a pinch of sea salt and stir.
2. Put the whisked egg in another bowl.
3. Dip chicken pieces in egg, then in coconut mixture, arrange them all on a lined baking sheet and bake at 350°F for 25 minutes.
4. Serve as a snack. Enjoy!

Nutrition:

- **Calories:** 330 kcal.
- **Protein:** 36.9 g.
- **Fat:** 13.6 g.
- **Carbohydrates:** 13.6 g.
- **Fiber:** 8.1 g.

34. Roasted Brussels Sprouts with Pecans and Gorgonzola

Preparation time: 10 minutes.

Cooking time: 35 minutes.

Servings: 4

Ingredients:

- 1 pound Brussels sprouts, fresh.
- ¼ c pecans, chopped.
- 1 tbsp olive oil.
- Extra olive oil to oil the baking tray.
- Pepper and salt for tasting.
- ¼ c. gorgonzola cheese. (If you prefer not to use the gorgonzola cheese, you can toss the Brussels sprouts when hot, with 2 tbsp butter instead.)

Directions:

1. Warm the oven to 350°F.
2. Rub a large pan or any vessel you wish to use with a little bit of olive oil. You can use a paper towel or a pastry brush.
3. Cut off the ends of the Brussels sprouts if you need to and then cut them in a lengthwise direction into halves. (Fear not if a few of the leaves come off of

them, some may become deliciously crunchy during cooking)

4. Chop up all of the pecans using a knife and then measure them for the amount.

5. Put your Brussels sprouts as well as the sliced pecans inside a bowl, and cover them all with some olive oil, pepper, and salt (be generous).

6. Arrange all of your pecans and Brussels sprouts onto your roasting pan in a single layer

7. Roast this for 30 to 35 minutes, or when they become tender and can be pierced with a fork easily. Stir during cooking if you wish to get a more even browning.

8. Once cooked, toss them with the gorgonzola cheese (or butter) before you serve them. Serve them hot.

Nutrition:

- **Calories:** 149 kcal.
- **Protein:** 5 g.
- **Fat:** 11 g.
- **Carbohydrates:** 10 g.
- **Fiber:** 4 g.

35. Artichoke Petals Bites

Preparation time: 10 minutes.

Cooking time: 10 minutes.

Servings: 8

Ingredients:

- 8 oz. artichoke petals, boiled, drained, without salt.
- ½ c. almond flour.
- 4 oz. Parmesan, grated.
- 2 tbsp almond butter, melted.

Directions:

1. In the mixing bowl, mix up together almond flour and grated Parmesan.
2. Preheat the oven to 355°F.
3. Dip the artichoke petals in the almond butter and then coat in the almond flour mixture.
4. Place them in the tray.
5. Transfer the tray to the preheated oven and cook the petals for 10 minutes.
6. Chill the cooked petal bites a little before serving.

Nutrition:

- **Calories:** 93 kcal.
- **Protein:** 6.54 g.
- **Fat:** 3.72 g.
- **Carbohydrates:** 9.08 g.

36. Stuffed Beef Loin in Sticky Sauce

Preparation time: 15 minutes.

Cooking time: 6 minutes.

Servings: 4

Ingredients:

- 1 tbsp erythritol.
- 1 tbsp lemon juice.
- 4 tbsp water.
- ½ tsp tomato sauce.
- ¼ tsp dried rosemary.
- 9 oz. beef loin.
- 3 oz. celery root, grated.
- 3 oz. bacon, sliced.
- 1 tbsp walnuts, chopped.
- ¾ tsp garlic, diced.
- 2 tsps butter.
- 1 tbsp olive oil.
- 1 tsp salt.
- ½ c. of water

Directions:

1. Cut the beef loin into the layer and spread it with the dried rosemary, butter, and salt. Then place over the beef loin grated celery root, sliced bacon, walnuts, and diced garlic.

2. Roll the beef loin and brush it with olive oil. Secure the meat with the help of the toothpicks. Place it in the tray and add ½ c. of water.

3. Cook the meat in the preheated to 365°F oven for 40 minutes.

Meanwhile, make the sticky sauce:

1. Mix up together erythritol, lemon juice, 4 tbsp of water, and butter.

2. Preheat the mixture until it starts to boil. Then add tomato sauce and whisk it well.

3. Bring the sauce to boil and remove from the heat.

4. When the beef loin is cooked, remove it from the oven and brush it with the cooked sticky sauce very generously.

5. Slice the beef roll and sprinkle with the remaining sauce.

37. Eggplant Fries

Preparation time: 10 minutes.

Cooking time: 15 minutes.

Servings: 8

Ingredients:

- 2 eggs.
- 2 c. almond flour.
- 2 tbsp coconut oil, spray.
- 2 eggplant, peeled and cut thinly.
- Salt and pepper.

Directions:

1. Preheat your oven to 400°F.
2. Take a bowl and mix with salt and black pepper in it
3. Take another bowl and beat eggs until frothy
4. Dip the eggplant pieces into eggs
5. Then coat them with a flour mixture
6. Add another layer of flour and egg
7. Then, take a baking sheet and grease with coconut oil on top
8. Bake for about 15 minutes
9. Serve and enjoy.

Nutrition:

- **Calories:** 212 kcal.
- **Protein:** 8.6 g.
- **Fat:** 15.8 g.
- **Carbohydrates:** 12.1 g.

38. Parmesan Crisps

Preparation time: 5 minutes.

Cooking time: 25 minutes.

Servings: 8

Ingredients:

- 1 tsp butter.
- 8 oz. Parmesan cheese, full fat and shredded.

Directions:

1. Preheat your oven to 400°F.
2. Put parchment paper on a baking sheet and grease with butter.
3. Spoon parmesan into 8 mounds, spreading them apart evenly.
4. Flatten them.
5. Bake for 5 minutes until browned.
6. Let them cool.
7. Serve and enjoy.

Nutrition:
- **Calories:** 133 kcal.
- **Protein:** 11 g.
- **Fat:** 11 g.
- **Carbohydrates:** 1g.

39. Roasted Broccoli

Preparation time: 5 minutes

Cooking time: 20 minutes

Servings: 4

Ingredients:

- 4 c. broccoli florets.
- 1 tbsp olive oil.
- Salt and pepper to taste.

Directions:

1. Preheat your oven to 400°F.
2. Add broccoli in a zip bag alongside oil and shake until coated.
3. Add seasoning and shake again.
4. Spread broccoli out on the baking sheet, bake for 20 minutes.
5. Let it cool and serve.

Nutrition:

- **Calories:** 62 kcal.
- **Protein:** 4 g.
- **Fat:** 4 g.
- **Carbohydrates:** 4 g.

40. Almond Flour Muffins

Preparation time: 15 minutes.

Cooking time: 30 minutes.

Servings: 8

Ingredients:

- 1/3 c. of pumpkin puree.
- 3 eggs.
- 1 c. almond flour
- 2 tbsp agave nectar.
- 2 tbsp coconut oil.
- 1 tsp vanilla extract.
- 1 tsp white vinegar.
- 1 c. chopped fruits.
- 1 tsp baking soda.
- ½ tsp salt.

Directions:

1. Preheat the oven to 350°F.
2. Line the muffin tin with paper liners

3. In the first mixing bowl, whisk the almond flour, salt, and baking soda.

4. In the second mixing bowl, whisk the pumpkin puree, eggs, coconut oil, agave nectar, vanilla extract, and vinegar.

5. Now add this puree mix of the second bowl to the first bowl and blend everything well.

6. Add the chopped fruits to the blend.

7. Pour the mixture into the muffin cups in your pan.

8. Bake for 15 to 20 minutes. Ensure that the contents have set in the center, and a golden-brown lining has started to appear at the edges.

9. Transfer the muffins to a cooling rack and let them cool completely.

Nutrition:

- **Calories:** 75 kcal.
- **Protein:** 0 g.
- **Fat:** 6 g.
- **Carbohydrates:** 4 g.

41. Apple Bread

Preparation time: 20 minutes.

Cooking time: 60 minutes.

Servings: 10

Ingredients:

- ½ c. honey.
- ½ tsp nutmeg.
- ½ tsp salt.
- 1 c. applesauce, sweetened.
- 1 tsp baking soda.
- 1 tsp vanilla extract.
- 2 ¼ c. whole wheat flour.
- 2 lg. eggs.
- 2 tbsp vegetable oil (or preferred oil).
- 2 tsps baking powder.
- 2 tsps cinnamon.
- 4 c. apples, diced.

Directions:

1. Preheat the oven to 375°F and oil a loaf pan with non-stick spray or your choice of oil.

2. In a large mixing bowl, beat eggs until completely smooth.

3. Add the honey, oil, applesauce, cinnamon, vanilla, nutmeg, baking powder, baking soda, and salt. Whisk until completely combined and smooth.

4. Add the flour into the bowl and whisk to combine, making sure not to over-mix. Simply stir it enough to incorporate the flour.

5. Add apples to the batter and mix once more to combine.

6. Pour the batter into the loaf pan and smooth the top with your spatula.

7. Bake for 60 minutes, or until an inserted toothpick in the center comes out clean.

8. Let stand for 10 minutes, then transfer the loaf to a cooling rack to cool completely.

9. Slice into 10 pieces and serve!

Nutrition:

- **Calories:** 210 kcal.
- **Protein:** 5 g.
- **Fat:** 5 g.
- **Carbohydrates:** 41 g.
- **Sugar:** 17 g.

42. Coconut Protein Balls

Preparation time: 20 minutes.

Cooking time: 0 minutes.

Servings: 27

Ingredients:

- ¼ c. dark chocolate chips.
- ½ c. coconut flakes, unsweetened.
- ½ c. water.
- 1 ½ c. almonds, raw & unsalted.
- 2 tbsp cocoa powder, unsweetened.
- 3 c. Medjool dates, pitted.
- 4 scoops whey protein powder, unsweetened.

Directions:

1. Process almonds in a food processor until flour is formed. Add the water and dates to the flour and continue to process until fully combined. You may need to stop intermittently to scrape down the sides of the bowl.

2. Add cocoa and protein to the processor and continue to process until well combined. You may need to stop intermittently to scrape down the sides of the bowl.

3. Pull the blade out of the processor (carefully!) and use your spatula to gather all of the dough in one place inside the processor container.

4. On a plate or in a large, shallow dish, spread the coconut flakes.

5. Using a spoon, scoop out a little bit of the dough at a time and roll it into balls, then roll each one in the coconut flakes.

6. Refrigerate for at least 30 min before enjoying.

These can be refrigerated for up to 1 week, or frozen for up to 3 months!

Nutrition:

- **Calories:** 108 kcal.
- **Protein:** 5 g.
- **Fat:** 4 g.
- **Carbohydrates:** 16 g.
- **Sugar:** 13 g.

Conclusion

Many people have found benefits from fasting, no matter their age. Women, in particular, may feel that they will not lose weight or be able to stick with the diet. They might even hear the criticism of other women who are doing it: "You're too old to be doing this!"

In reality, intermittent fasting can help you lose weight, have more energy, and gain a better connection with your body. Women over the age of 60 find it easier to fast than men of the same age because they have a lower risk of health complications and do not lose as much muscle mass while fasting as men do. There are two different forms of intermittent fasting known as the 16/8 method and the 5/2 method.

In the 16/8 method, you fast for 16 hours and then only eat for 8 hours. You can break up the fasting period any way that works best for your schedule. For example, you could choose to stop eating at 8 p.m. and start eating again at 12 p.m. This will require a lot of discipline at first because it is hard to go that long without food! In the 5/2 method, you fast for 2 days a week. For example, you would eat whatever you wanted on Monday and then eat very little on Tuesday and Wednesday.

If you're just getting started with intermittent fasting, this is a great place to start. To stay within your recommended daily intake, you should keep track of your calories even when you aren't eating.

The key is to eat as little as possible on non-fasting days so that your body can burn fat while you sleep without having to worry about digestion. You should drink lots of water before bed to help with sleep and dehydration. 5 days out of the week, it is recommended that you consume carbohydrates after exercising or at night before going to bed in order to replenish muscle glycogen.

Another benefit of this method is that it can help women with irregular cycles have more regular periods. However, if you are going to try this method, slowly transition to it starting on the day of the fast. By taking the first 24 hours off from eating in order to begin with, you will be able to better regulate your period so that it doesn't become irregular.

A lot of people say that this should only be done once or twice a year, but for some women, it can work year-round because the effect is cumulative on your metabolism. After about 3 months of fasting, many women will start losing at least 10 pounds.

When you cut calories, your body will start to consume adipose tissue. You should be prepared for a reduction in energy levels because this is the time where women will start to feel hungry. Just remember that you aren't doing this so that you can eat a lot; you are doing it so that you can be healthy and lose weight.

As soon as enough adipose tissue has been burned off, you will notice an improvement in your energy levels and endurance. During the fast, try to move around for at least 20 minutes a day, but do not exercise because that will break the fast too quickly. Yoga is usually the best exercise for women who are just starting out with fasting since it doesn't involve doing anything too vigorous.

Your body will start to adapt to eating less beginning on day eight of fasting. Once your body has adjusted, you should be able to maintain your weight loss and have healthy periods.

BOOK 2
KETO FOR WOMAN OVER 50

The Complete Guide to the Ketogenic Diet for Senior Women, Including the Basics, 120 recipes, and 30-Day Weight Loss Plans for Beginners, Complete With a 30-Day Meal Plan and Physical Exercises to Maintain Ketosis

SHANA KATHY

Introduction

At some point, we have all come across the phrase, "You are what you eat." But is this the case? And if it is the case, what exactly should we be putting in our mouths to maintain a healthy lifestyle? Well, many nutritionists would argue that there is the truth behind this saying. In other words, what we eat matters. It matters so much that our health depends upon us making healthy choices regarding our diets. This is, even more, the case for the elderly. It has become common knowledge that a poor diet leads to obesity and makes us susceptible to chronic diseases. The good news is that this does not have to be your story. The ketogenic diet (also known as the keto diet) is a low-carb, high-fat diet that has been found to not only improve health, but prevent diseases like diabetes, cancer, epilepsy, and Alzheimer's. This is fantastic news, wouldn't you say? The keto diet helps you to lose weight quickly, improve your health, require fewer visits to the doctor, and, ultimately, prolongs your life.

So, how does it work? Well, the goal of the keto diet is to help your body to burn down your fat reserves. Therefore, the ketogenic diet helps your body to enter this process by putting it into a state called 'ketosis.' Under normal circumstances, your body would naturally burn down the carbohydrates that you eat to use as energy. However, since the keto diet restricts your carb intake, your body goes into a metabolic state of ketosis, burning your stored fat instead. There is no need to be alarmed, ketosis is a natural process that happens all the time. In this case, however, your body remains in ketosis for a longer period, ensuring that your weight slips off drastically. The goal is to get your body to create ketones from your stored fat cells (hence the name ketogenic diet), which your body will use as energy.

Also, when on the diet, it will be helpful for you to track your macronutrients. Tracking your macronutrient intake will help you to hit your dietary goals faster. Macronutrients are fats, proteins, and carbohydrates. Tracking them simply means knowing how much you are consuming.

This will ensure that you are adhering to your diet, and help you to lose weight faster and more consistently. First, you will need to determine how much energy your unique day-to-day activities require so that will not strain your body. If you are more active in your day, you will need to have more protein and a few more carbs.

With that said, I can promise you that you will not regret reading this book. This book has all you will ever need to know about adopting a ketogenic diet. I aim to give you all the tools that you need to make your ketogenic diet journey a success. Included in the book are a variety of delicious recipes that will keep your taste buds satisfied, which will make sure that you do not cheat on your diet. These are recipes for breakfast, lunch, and supper (and even snacks in between). Variety is the key component in adhering to this diet. If you eat the same thing every day, you are bound to fall off your diet. Therefore, the book also includes a shopping list that will make sure that you have all the goodies you need for these recipes. Furthermore, a portion of the book will help you to customize your diet to suit your unique tastes. All these are but a few of what this book offers, so let us not waste any more time, and jump right in.

Chapter 1: What You Need to Know About the Ketogenic Diet

The ketogenic diet is not a new concept. It has been used for its medicinal benefits for about 100 years. Around 500 B.C, fasting was used to treat illnesses like epilepsy and seizures. Recently, researchers developed the ketogenic diet which not only resembles the fasting diets of ancient times but treats the same diseases (i.e., epilepsy, seizures, Alzheimer's, diabetes, and cancer). William Lennox, from the Harvard Medical School, noticed that seizures began to subside 2–3 days into fasting and concluded that this was due to a change in metabolism, or rather a change in the fuel that the body was using (Arnold, 2019). The noted change in fuel is from glycogen to fat. You see, your body can function on different sources of fuel. There are three different fuel sources, to be exact: glucose (from carbohydrates), fatty acids (from dietary fats), and proteins. Your body is naturally inclined to use glucose as energy because it is easier to absorb and store as fat. When you are on a ketogenic diet, your body is encouraged to break down fat into ketones and use those as fuel instead of glucose. As mentioned earlier, the primary goal of the ketogenic diet is to keep your body under a state of 'ketosis.' "Ketosis is a metabolic state, in which the body has shifted from using glucose as the primary fuel source for supplying its energy demands with ketone bodies" (Land, 2017). Ketosis can be achieved by following a low-carb diet for about three days.

There is a range of amazing benefits that come with following the ketogenic diet. If you are new to this concept, you might be skeptical, even wary that you will thrive on this diet. However, your body will function better fueling on ketones than it does on glucose. If you think about it, periods of fasting were normal for our human ancestors. Moreover, innumerable dieters have experienced improved health by decreasing their intake of sugar and carbs and embarking on keto-based diets. Here are a few interesting facts about ketosis:

- Ketones produce more energy than glucose.
- Glucose metabolism creates oxidative stress which speeds up aging.
- Under ketosis, it is easier to burn stored fat and this leads to drastic weight loss.
- Fueling on ketones clears your mind because you are less obsessed with your next treat.

Now, I am sure that you are asking yourself what you can and cannot eat on this diet. First, I would like to say that this diet is not as restrictive as you would think. If you fill your pantry with a variety of good things, the keto diet will not feel like a burden. Let's start with the things you can eat. You can only include low-carb foods like leafy greens, chicken, beef, eggs, a little diary, nuts, olive oil, butter, and seeds. Make sure that you stay away from high-carb foods like sugar, grains, fruit, potatoes, vegetable oils, and processed meats. This list is not exhaustive. I will go into further detail later in the book.

How to Track Macronutrients

Although all the foods noted above are compatible with the keto diet, you need to know how much of each you should eat. You cannot munch on many of these foods to excess and expect to get great results. This is why you need to track the intake of your macronutrients. Tracking macronutrients is not just to ensure that you lose weight, but it is also a good tool to make sure that you do not starve yourself. You can make use of various online macronutrient calculators that can help you adjust your diet to your unique lifestyle. These calculators are important because the good ones calculate your level of activity as well. Nevertheless, the standard breakdown of daily macronutrient percentages is as follows:

- 5–10% carbs (30–50 g NET)
- 15–30% protein (0,6–1,0 g / lb)
- 70–80% fat

Ketosis

You will transition into ketosis three days into a ketogenic diet if you have been tracking your macronutrients well. It is helpful to know how to identify when you are in a state of ketosis.

Keto Breath

When you enter into ketosis, your breath begins to swell noticeably. The breaking down of fats by your liver releases acetone. This acetone is responsible for the change in your breath. Keto breath smells fruity, and/or metallic; many have likened it to the smell of overripe apples. You will find that you cannot get rid of the odor by brushing your teeth or using mouthwash. However, as the weeks progress, the smell will subside.

Thirst and a Dry Mouth

When your body is under ketosis, you will notice that you will become thirsty and experience a dry mouth. Under ketosis, your body has an increased need for water. You will also notice that you will urinate more and the urine will have a pungent smell.

Appetite Loss

The longer you adhere to the diet, the more opportunity you give your body to tap into your fat reserves for energy. Ultimately, this will result in decreased cravings for food. Your body will rely on your body's fat for sustenance so you will not need to eat as much as you used to. This effect of the diet is quite helpful to the whole process because, if you are disciplined, your body will also come on board to help you succeed. You will also experience increased energy. Contrary to what you may be thinking, you will not feel starved and listless. You will realize that your mind functions better on this diet. You will have a clearer headspace, which will lead to a better mood.

Blood Tests and Urine Tests

Blood and urine tests are the most accurate ways to detect whether you are in ketosis. The go-to test, however, is the urine test because it is inexpensive and you can do it at home. All you need to do is purchase the strips at a health store, dip a strip into a urine sample, and wait 15 seconds to get a color spectrum result. The spectrum will indicate how deep into ketosis you are. The darker the color, the deeper you are into ketosis.

How to Maintain Ketosis

This diet relies on you building a pattern that works for your body and your day-to-day activities. It will help a great deal if, when you do reach a ketogenic state, you can stay in it for a prolonged period. Fluctuating in and out of a ketogenic diet will exhaust you, and lead you to feel that you cannot keep up. Therefore, you need to commit to maintaining ketosis. Ketosis should become a new normal for your body. Subsequently, you need to learn to identify when you are and are not in ketosis so that you can control the process.

First, you need to go into this diet aggressively. This is why it is important to be prepared, to make sure that you have all that you need to commit to the diet. Starting strong will cause a drastic change in the way your body functions. Therefore, you will be better able to notice the key signs of ketosis. If you were hoping to wean yourself slowly off of carbs, chuck this idea. Once you have started keto, you need to concern yourself with maintaining the momentum. Of course, this requires discipline. However, getting rid of the temptations in your pantry can help. Also, notice that the prescribed shopping lists contain a variety of delicious foods from which to choose: this should make your life better. The more variety, the less likely you are to get bored with the diet. So ensure that you create shopping lists with a lot of variety and buy products with many different flavors.

Testing your ketone level will also help you to maintain ketosis. When you know you are in it, you are more likely to maintain it. So, you might need to invest in ketone testing strips. Once you have used the strips long enough, you will be able to feel when you are or are not in ketosis; at this point, you can stop purchasing the strips.

Furthermore, tracking your macronutrient intake (as explained above) will ensure that you are in ketosis for long periods. Obviously, if you are eating the correct ratio for your individual needs every day, you will be able to stay in ketosis longer. When you have a meal that is a little bit high on carbs, then you need to compensate by being active.

Tips to Achieve Keto Success for Beginners

The key to keto success is getting into a disciplined eating regime that tracks what you eat and your energy output. In order to do this, you need to follow the true keto diet. Although you can work around your diet to suit your lifestyle, keto success requires that you stick to a macronutrient ratio for eating. You may be tempted to cheat, but doing so will cause you to fluctuate in and out of ketosis which, in turn, will exhaust you. The body thrives on predictability. When you cheat, you throw your body off. In other words, you want to commit to the diet before you begin. Ask yourself what you have to gain if you succeed at this diet. Use these goals to keep you going. Make sure that your goals are attainable, and create a realistic timeline to achieve them.

Try to adopt keto as a new lifestyle. By this, I mean that you should make it enjoyable. It should not feel like torture. With the recipes provided in this book, you have a variety to make sure that you do not get tired of the diet. And, as mentioned before, you need to design your macronutrient tracking according to your body's specific demands. Starving yourself in hopes of attaining faster results will not work.

Work with your body by staying hydrated. When under ketosis, you will urinate more than usual. This means you will lose a lot of water and electrolytes. The body will be trying to flush the stored glucose from your body. Help your body to cope with this new system by staying hydrated. You can add salt to your water to get electrolytes back into the system or you can buy electrolyte minerals.

A new trend in dieting is to merge the keto diet with intermittent fasting. This is not necessary but it can help you attain your results faster. Fasting will get you into ketosis faster. And, of course, as with any other diet, getting some activity into your day will hasten the process. Start with a simple exercise, then move towards an intensity that you can manage. Be careful not to overdo it. Remember, you are already on a low-calorie diet.

Last, keep your stress levels low and get enough sleep. Adopt stress reduction techniques like yoga, journaling, or talking about your feelings. The stress hormone cortisol can affect the hormones that are responsible for weight gain. If you are under stress and start keto, you may not experience the expected results. On the other hand, help your body to recharge by making sure that you have a good night's sleep. Limit screen time and do not drink stimulating drinks before sleeping.

How to Counter the Hormonal Change Affecting Metabolism

There are about nine hormones that are known to control weight. They influence our appetites and how much fat we store. But you can control the way these hormones affect your weight.

Insulin

Insulin is produced by the beta cells of the pancreas. It helps our metabolism by depressing blood glucose levels. Our bodies need insulin because, when our bodies are insulin resistant, our blood sugar levels are always high and this can

lead to health problems, like obesity and diabetes. Overeating things that contain lots of sugar and carbohydrates can lead to insulin resistance. To mitigate this, here are a few things you can do:
- Minimize sugar
- Reduce carbohydrates
- Eat lots of protein
- Eat healthy fats
- Drink green tea
- Get enough magnesium
- Exercise regularly

Leptin

Leptin is a hormone that is secreted by our fat cells. It gives us that feeling of fullness when we eat a lot of food. Hence, it is responsible for reducing our appetites and tells us when we have had enough. Without it, we would overeat and, more than likely, become overweight. This is because leptin tells the brain when enough fat has been stored so that we will stop eating. But since leptin is produced by fat cells, why do obese people eat too much food? People with more fat cells have relatively higher leptin levels; however, it does not always work as it should and that phenomenon is called leptin resistance. There are a few ways to improve leptin sensitivity:
- Avoid inflammatory foods
- Eat anti-inflammatory foods like fatty fish
- Exercise regularly
- Get enough sleep

Ghrelin

Ghrelin is the hunger hormone. When our stomach is empty, it releases ghrelin that tells the hypothalamus that you need to eat. Ghrelin is high before eating and lowest after we've had a meal. However, studies show that ghrelin decreases slightly in obese people after they have had a meal. You can improve its function by:
- Avoiding sugar
- Eating protein at every meal

Chapter 2: Basic Items That Should Be in Your Pantry (or on Your Shopping List)

Meats and Poultry:
- Chicken, whole or parts
- Ground turkey
- Beef steaks and tips
- Beef or pork roasts
- Ground beef
- Bacon, ham, and pork sausage
- Pork loin, chops, or steaks
- Pork or beef ribs
- Turkey and ham cold cuts

Seafood
- Fresh or frozen shrimp
- Fresh or frozen fish
- Fresh or frozen scallops
- Canned tuna or salmon in oil or water
- Crab

Dairy
- Heavy cream
- Sour cream
- Cream cheese
- Butter
- Cheeses
- Full-fat Greek yogurt, plain
- Eggs

Vegetables
- Bell peppers
- Broccoli
- Cucumbers
- Cabbage
- Cauliflower
- Lettuce (preferably varieties with large leaves, like romaine)
- Leafy green vegetables, like spinach and kale
- Onions
- Garlic
- Squash and zucchini
- Mushrooms
- Artichoke hearts
- Asparagus
- Bok Choy
- Garlic
- Onion
- Fruit (enjoy once weight and health are stabilized)
- Blueberries

Fruit (enjoy once weight and health are stabilized)
- Blueberries
- Blackberries
- Raspberries
- Cranberries
- Strawberries

Nuts and Seeds
- Pumpkin seeds
- Pecans
- Hazelnuts
- Walnuts
- Macadamias
- Sunflower seeds

- Sesame seeds
- Almonds

Cooking and Baking
- Chicken and vegetable stock
- Whey protein powder
- Splenda or other artificial sweeteners (I prefer stevia)
- Your favorite extracts (vanilla, almond, lemon, peppermint)
- Broth or bouillon
- Unsweetened cocoa powder
- Plain gelatin
- Xanthan gum
- Extra-virgin olive oil
- Coconut oil
- Sesame oil
- Almond flour or other nut flours

Miscellaneous
- Lemon and lime juice
- Mayonnaise
- Beef jerky or beef sticks
- Unsweetened almond milk
- Nut kinds of butter
- Raspberries
- Strawberries
- Blackberries
- Hazelnuts
- Nuts and Seeds
- Cranberries
- Almonds
- Pecans
- Walnuts
- Macadamias
- Sunflower seeds

- Pumpkin seeds
- Sesame seeds
- Cooking and Baking
- Chicken and vegetable stock
- Whey protein powder
- Your favorite extracts (vanilla, almond, lemon, peppermint)
- Broth or bouillon
- Unsweetened cocoa powder
- Plain gelatin
- Xanthan gum
- Extra-virgin olive oil
- Coconut oil
- Sesame oil
- Almond flour or other nut flours
- Miscellaneous
- Lemon and lime juice
- Mayonnaise
- Beef jerky or beef sticks
- Unsweetened almond milk
- Nut kinds of butter
- Flax Meal
- Olives
- Pickles
- Herbs and spices
- Pork rinds (crushed pork rinds are a wonderful bread crumb substitute)
- Salsa
- Hot sauce

Chapter 3: Keto Recipes for Breakfast

Keto Breakfast Recipes

Breakfast Detox Tea

Time: 5 minutes
Serving Size: 1 serving
Prep Time: 5 minutes
Nutritional Facts/Info:
Calories 84
Carbs 20.2 g
Fat 0.3 g
Protein 0.4 g
Ingredients:
- 8 oz of warm water
- 1 tbsp of honey
- 1 tsp of cinnamon
- 2 tbsps of lemon juice
- 1 dash of cayenne
- 2 tbsps of apple cider vinegar

Directions:
1. Add all the ingredients together into a mug and stir well
2. Serve and enjoy!

Egg White Spinach Omelet

Time: 30 minutes
Serving Size: 1 serving
Prep Time: 15 minutes
Cook Time: 15 minutes
Nutritional Facts/Info:
Calories 203
Carbs 18 g
Fat 5 g
Protein 20 g
Ingredients:
- 1 egg yolk
- 4–5 egg whites
- ½ or 1 tomato
- 2 tbsp (30 ml), coconut, almond, or soy milk
- 1 handful shredded spinach
- 1 tbsp onion
- 1 pinch preferred herb olive oil cooking spray

Directions:
1. Chop the vegetables
2. Beat the eggs, mixing the yolks and egg whites.
3. Add coconut milk to the eggs and beat the mixture.
4. Put some oil into a pan and fry the vegetables till they are tender.
5. Set the vegetables aside, oil the pan again, put the stove on medium heat, and pour the eggs.
6. Cook until the eggs are firm.
7. Place the vegetables on one side and fold the side of the egg over them.

Keto Waffles

Time: 30 minutes
Serving Size: 5 servings

Prep Time: 30 minutes

Cook Time: 4–5 minutes

Nutritional Facts/Info:

Calories 256 | Carbs 1.3 g | Fat 25.5 g | Protein 5.8 g

Ingredients:

- 5 eggs (separated)
- 1 tsp of baking powder
- 4 tbsp of coconut flour
- 2 tips of vanilla
- 5 tbsps of granulated sweetener
- 4 1/2 oz of melted butter
- 3 tbsps of full-fat milk or cream

Directions:

1. Use one bowl to whisk your egg whites till they become firm and you can see peaks forming.
2. Use a second bowl to mix the egg yolks, sweetener, baking powder, and coconut flour.

3. Add the melted butter into the mixture in the second bowl, slowly mixing everything till it is well incorporated.
4. Add milk and vanilla into the second bowl, and mix everything slowly.
5. Gently fold the whisked egg whites into the mixture, making sure that you keep as much air in the mixture as possible.
6. Place the waffle mixture into a warm waffle maker and cook until golden.
7. Continue to use the mixture till it is finished.
8. Serve and enjoy!

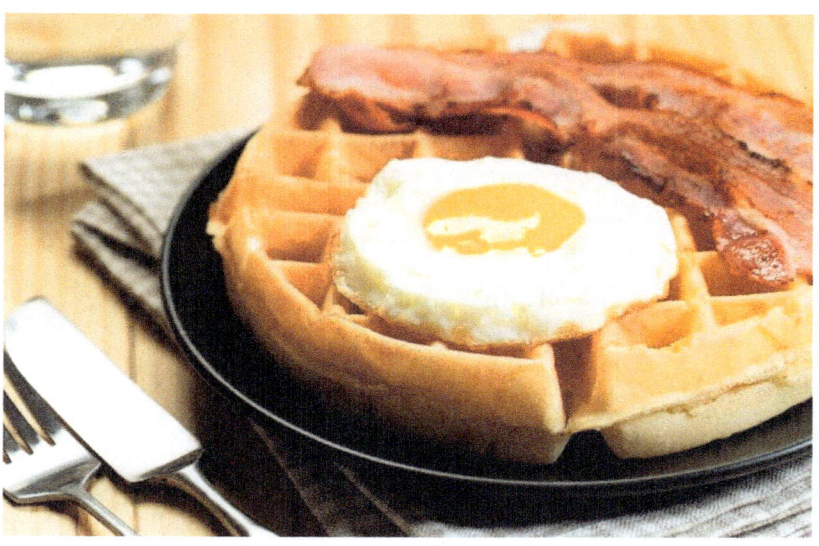

Bacon Frittata

Time: 25 minutes
Serving Size: 6 slices
Prep Time: 5 minutes
Cook Time: 20 minutes
Nutritional Facts/Info:
Calories 408
Carbs 2.4 g
Fat 31 g
Protein 9.2 g

Ingredients:
- 7 bacon slices
- 1 tbsp olive oil
- 4 large mushroom caps
- 4 oz fresh chopped asparagus
- 4 oz fresh cubed mozzarella cheese
- 1 medium green bell pepper
- 8–9 large eggs
- 2 oz grated goat cheese
- 2 oz heavy cream
- 2 oz grated parmesan cheese
- Salt & pepper to taste

Directions:
1. Chop the green bell pepper, bacon, asparagus, and mushrooms roughly. Cube the mozzarella and then put it aside.
2. Preheat the oven to 350°F.
3. Sprinkle some olive oil into a hot pan. Once the oil in the pan is hot, add the chopped bacon.
4. Cook the bacon until it is brown. Then add the green pepper and allow it to cook with the bacon fat till it is soft.

5. On the other side, add eggs, heavy cream, parmesan cheese, and black pepper into a container. Mix the eggs well with a whisk.
6. When the green pepper softens, add the mushrooms, and stir well. The mushrooms should soak in the fat.
7. Add the fresh asparagus to the pan. Leave it to cook for a while, then sprinkle the mozzarella cheese on top.
8. Then, pour eggs over onto them. Get the eggs under and around the ingredients in the pan by using a spoon or a spatula to lift the ingredients from the pan's bottom.
9. Add grated goat cheese over the top. Put the mixture in the oven for about 8 minutes. Grill the top in the grill for 4–6 minutes more.
10. Use a spoon to remove from the oven, and pry the frittata edges away from the pan.
11. Flip out of the pan and slice, serve and enjoy!

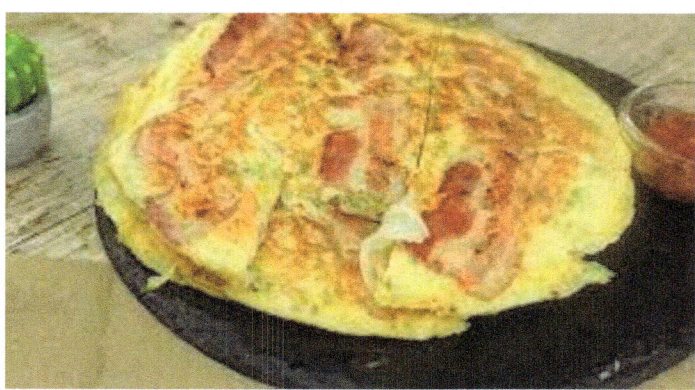

Cheese & Onion Quiche

Time: 50 minutes
Serving Size: 2 quiches
Prep Time: 10 minutes
Cook Time: 20–25 minutes
Nutritional Facts/Info:
Calories 382
Carbs 7 g
Fat 33 g
Protein 16 g

Ingredients:
- 40 oz shredded Colby Jack cheese and/or Muenster, divided
- 2 tbsp butter plus more
- 12 large eggs
- 16 oz heavy cream
- 1 large white onion, finely chopped
- 2 tsp dried thyme
- 1 tsp ground black pepper
- 1 tsp salt

Directions:
1. Turn the oven on to 350°F and allow it to heat up. Then add the butter to a skillet and melt it over medium heat.
2. Add all of the vegetables into the skillet, fry till the onions are soft and translucent. Then remove them from the heat and leave them to cool.
3. Butter 2 quiche pans or deep pie pans of 10-inch. Then, put 2 cups of Muenster or shredded cheese at the bottom of the buttered pans.
4. Add half of the cooled vegetables to each pan.
5. Crack some eggs into a large mixing bowl. Then, add the cream and spices, beating everything together till thoroughly mixed and frothy.

6. Pour half of the mixture of eggs, cream, and spices over each pan of veggies and cheese. Then, gently add cheese and vegetables evenly into egg and cream using a fork.
7. Place the quiche pans into the oven, leaving 1 inch of space between the pans. Bake for 20–25 minutes, until it is set and puffy and golden in the center.
8. Slice the quiche, server, and enjoy!

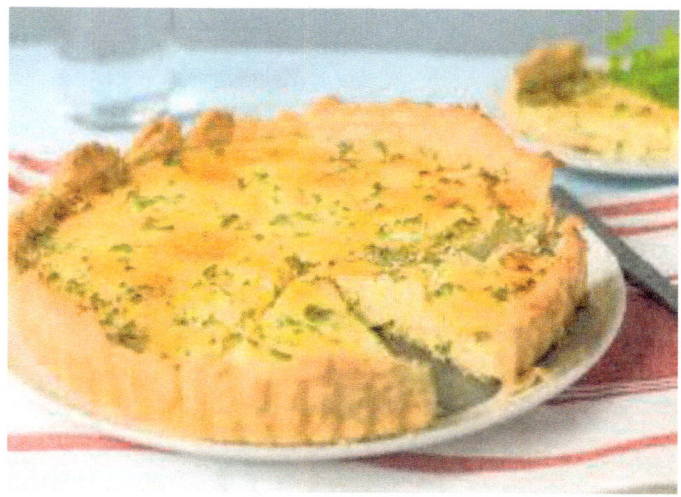

Keto French Toast

Time: 20 minutes
Serving Size: 4 muffins
Prep Time: 10 minutes
Cook Time: 10 minutes
Nutritional Facts/Info:
Calories 345
Carbs 7.8 g
Fat 29.4 g
Protein 14.2 g
Ingredients:
- 8 large eggs
- 2 tsp of baking powder
- 26 oz of unsweetened almond milk
- 10 oz of coconut flour
- 1 tbsp of Swerve or sugar equivalent
- 10 oz of melted butter
- 1 tsp of vanilla extract
- 10 oz of fresh whole butter
- 4 oz of heavy whipping cream
- 2 g of salt

Directions:
1. Mix the baking powder, baking powder, salt, and sugar.
2. In another bowl, beat together 4 of your 8 eggs. Then, add 1/4 cup of your almond milk and vanilla. Mix everything.
3. Add the dry and wet ingredients together, and mix. Do this as you pour in the melted butter.
4. Spray 12 microwave-safe containers with oil. Use wide containers.
5. Microwave the muffins for about six minutes. For each additional muffin add a minute to microwave time.

6. While the muffins are cooking, use a large-sized mixing bowl to whisk together your other 4 eggs, 1/2 cup of heavy cream, and 1/2 cup of almond milk.
7. Take the muffins out of the microwave, pop them out of the containers and allow them to cool for a minute. When they have cooled, add them to the egg mixture and leave them for a few minutes, allowing the flavors to blend and meld together. Toss them around in the mixture occasionally while letting them sit.
8. Once they've absorbed some of the mixtures, heat your large-sized frying pan over medium-low heat. Add some fresh butter and melt it.
9. Fry your muffins like you would French toast.
10. Serve and enjoy!

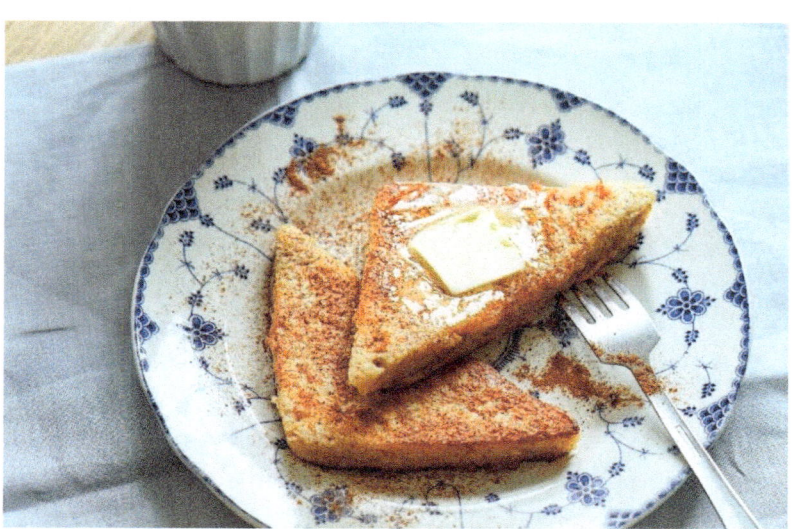

Crunchy Keto Cereal with Strawberries

Time: 10 minutes
Serving Size: 1

Prep Time: 5 minutes

Cook Time: 5 minutes

Nutritional Facts/Info:

Calories 192

Carbs 9.7 g

Fat 18.1 g

Protein 2.3 g

Ingredients:
- 1 package of Bob's Red Mill Flaked Coconut
- cinnamon
- stevia
- unsweetened coconut almond milk
- 2 medium strawberries
- parchment paper/coconut oil

Directions:
1. Set the oven to 350°F and leave it to heat up fully.
2. Prepare the cookie tray with parchment paper. If you don't have parchment paper, grease your cooking sheet with coconut oil.
3. Distribute the coconut flakes to your cookie tray.
4. Place them in your oven for approximately 5 minutes.
5. Toss the flakes around and continue cooking till they are lightly toasted and light tan.
6. Take them out of the oven.
7. Sprinkle them lightly with cinnamon, and stevia.
8. Toss them into your bowl and pour your almond milk over them.
9. Slice up 2 strawberries as the garnish on top.
10. Serve and enjoy!

Homemade Sage Sausage Patties

Time: 25 minutes
Serving Size: 8 servings

Prep Time: 10 minutes

Cook Time: 15 minutes

Nutritional Facts/Info:

Calories 162

Carbs 1 g

Fat 11 g

Protein 13 g

Ingredients:
- 1 lb ground pork
- 26 oz shredded cheddar cheese
- 2 oz buttermilk
- 1 tbsp finely chopped onion
- 2 tsp rubbed sage
- 3/4 tsp salt
- 3/4 tsp pepper
- 1/8 tsp dried oregano
- 1/8 tsp garlic powder

Directions:
1. Use a bowl to combine all ingredients.
2. Mix them all, lightly but thoroughly.
3. Shape the mixture into eight ½ inch thick patties.
4. Put them in the refrigerator for 1 hour.
5. Fry them in a large cast-iron or other heavy skillet.
6. Let them cook over medium heat until a thermometer reads 160 degrees Fahrenheit.
7. Flipping them over for about 6–8 minutes on each side.

Cinnamon Roll Cereal

Time: 20 minutes
Serving Size: 4 servings

Prep Time: 10 minutes

Cook Time: 10 minutes

Nutritional Facts/Info:

Calories 753

Carbs 29.5 g

Fat 75.1 g

Protein 9.5 g

Ingredients:
- 1 cup crushed pecans
- 1/3 cup chia seed
- ½ cup cauliflower, riced
- 3 ½ cups coconut milk
- 3 oz cream cheese
- 1/3 cup flax seed
- 3 tbsp butter
- 1 ½ tsp cinnamon
- 1/2 tsp vanilla
- 1/4 cup heavy cream
- 1 tsp maple flavor
- 1/4 tsp nutmeg

- 1/4 tsp allspice
- 10–15 drops liquid stevia
- 3 tbsp erythritol, powdered

Directions:
1. Crumble the cauliflower in the food processor to form a rice-like consistency and then set aside.
2. Then start to heat the coconut milk.
3. Use a skillet over medium heat and crush the pecans; add them to the skillet to toast over low heat.
4. Add the cauliflower to the coconut milk and bring it to a boil.
5. Then reduce to a simmer, and add the spices and combine.
6. Grind the erythritol and add it to the skillet.
7. Now add the chia seed, stevia, and flax. Mix everything thoroughly.
8. Lastly, add butter, cream cheese, and cream to the skillet and mix again. If desired, add xanthan gum to make it a bit thicker.

Eggs Florentine Casserole

Time: 50 min
Serving Size: 12 servings

Prep Time: 20 min

Cook Time: 30 min

Nutritional Facts/Info:

Calories 271

Carbs 6 g

Fat 20 g

Protein 16 g

Ingredients:
- 1 lb bulk pork sausage
- 2 tbsp butter
- 1 large onion, chopped
- 1 cup sliced fresh mushrooms
- 1 10 oz package frozen spinach, chopped, thawed, and then squeezed dry
- 12 large eggs
- 2 cups 2% milk
- 1 cup shredded Swiss cheese
- 1 cup shredded sharp cheddar cheese
- 1/4 tsp paprika

Directions:
1. First, turn up the oven to reach 350°F.
2. Using a large skillet, cook the sausage over medium heat until it is no longer pink, this should take about 6–8 minutes.
3. Break it into crumbles, then drain and transfer to a 13" x 9" inch pre-greased baking dish.
4. Now use the same skillet to heat butter over medium-high heat and add onion and mushrooms. Cook these and stir for 3–5 minutes or until tender.
5. Add spinach to the skillet, then scoop the vegetable mixture over sausage.
6. Use a large bowl to whisk eggs and milk until blended, then pour egg mixture over vegetables.
7. Sprinkle with cheeses and paprika.
8. Bake uncovered for 30–35 minutes until a thermometer reads 165° when inserted in the center. Check that the center is no longer runny by poking it with a fork and seeing if the fork comes out dry.
9. Allow it to stand 10 minutes before serving.

Keto Breakfast Grits

Time: 30 minutes
Serving Size: 2 servings

Prep Time: 15 minutes

Cook Time: 15 minutes

Nutritional Facts/Info:

Calories 484

Carbs 8.1 g

Fat 43.1 g

Protein 17.8 g

Ingredients:
- 2 tbsp butter
- 1/4 cup hemp hearts
- 2 cup cauliflower rice
- 1/4 tsp garlic powder
- 4 oz cremini mushrooms
- 1 cup almond milk
- 2 oz cheddar cheese
- Salt and pepper to taste
- 1/4 cup heavy cream

Directions:
1. Gather and prepare all ingredients.
2. Put 2 pans over medium heat on the stove. Then place half of the butter in each pan.
3. Pour the rice, cauliflower, and hemp hearts into a pan, mixing well before sautéing for roughly 3 minutes.
4. Fry the mushrooms in a new pan for 2–3 minutes, then season the mushrooms with salt and pepper and set them aside.
5. Add the garlic powder, heavy cream, salt and pepper, and almond milk to the cauliflower rice. Then stir well.
6. Lower the heat of the stove to medium-low, allow everything to simmer until the mixture is thick.
7. Be sure to add a touch of almond milk while it cooks should there be a need to prevent burning.
8. Turn off the stove and stir in half the shredded cheese.
9. Top everything with the fried mushrooms and the remaining shredded cheddar cheese.
10. Serve, and enjoy!

Keto Mushroom Omelet

Time: 30 minutes
Serving Size: 1 serving

Prep Time: 15 minutes

Cook Time: 15 minutes

Nutritional Facts/Info:

Calories 586

Carbs 6.9 g

Fat 48.2 g

Protein 29.7 g

Ingredients:
- 3 large egg
- 1 oz cheddar cheese, shredded
- 2 tbsp butter
- 80-gram cremini mushroom, sliced
- 1/4 medium red onion, diced
- salt and pepper to taste

Directions:
1. Shred the cheese, chop the onion, and slice the mushrooms.
2. Crack the eggs into a bowl and season with salt and pepper to your liking. Create a slightly frothy mix by beating the combined egg and seasoning with a fork.
3. Use a frying pan to melt the butter.
4. Once it has melted, toss in the prepared onion and mushrooms.
5. Season to taste, and cook the mushrooms until they are tender, stirring occasionally.
6. Drizzle the egg mixture into the pan covering the vegetables completely so it oozes through the gaps.
7. Once the sides begin to look cooked or start curling upwards and the top is still runny, sprinkle the cheddar cheese over the top
8. Carefully slide the spatula under the omelet before slowly folding it in half.
9. After a few minutes slowly lift a corner of the omelet and if you glimpse a crispy golden color, then it's ready to be taken out.
10. Serve, and enjoy!

Keto Lemon Chia Pudding

Time: 5 hours 10 minutes
Serving Size: 4 servings

Prep Time: 10 minutes

Cook Time: 5 hours

Nutritional Facts/Info:

Calories 343

Carbs 5.9 g

Fat 30.8 g

Protein 6.4 g

Ingredients:
- 1 cup canned coconut milk
- 1 cup unsweetened almond milk
- 1/2 cup heavy cream
- 1/2 cup chia seeds
- 3 tbsp stevia/erythritol blend
- 2 tsp lemon zest
- 1/2 cup lemon juice

Directions:
1. Put the coconut milk, cream, chia seeds, lemon juice, almond milk, stevia/erythritol blend, and lemon zest into a blender.
2. Mix it well using the pulse function on the blender until the flavors have combined.
3. Pour the pudding mixture into cups.
4. Place some plastic wrap over the cups to create an airtight seal before allowing them to harden for up to 5 hours in the refrigerator before enjoying.

Keto Crepes

Time: 20 minutes
Serving Size: 4 servings

Prep Time: 10 minutes

Cook Time: 10 minutes

Nutritional Facts/Info:

Calories 297

Carbs 3.7 g

Fat 25.2 g

Protein 12.6 g

Ingredients:
- 4 oz cream cheese, softened
- 3/4 cup almond flour
- 4 large eggs
- 1/4 cup unsweetened almond milk
- 2 tsp stevia erythritol blend

Directions:
1. Add all ingredients to a blender, and pulse until everything is smooth and well combined. Then let the mixture rest for a few minutes.
2. Place a non-stick pan over medium-low heat, and create a non-stick layer using cooking spray over the base of the dish.
3. Once the oil is hot, drizzle in up to 2 tbsp of batter, depending on how thick or thin you would like your crepe.
4. Swivel the pan to evenly spread out the batter, creating a thin layer.
5. Once the edges start to curl up slightly hardened, and the bottom can be loosened with a spatula. Flip it over, using a spatula, and allow it to cook evenly on the other side. When it is crisp and golden-brown, you will know it's ready.
6. Repeat this process with all of the batters.
7. Fill or top with your favorite fillings.
8. Serve warm and enjoy!

Keto Eggs Benedict

Time: 25 minutes
Serving Size: 2 servings

Prep Time: 10 minutes

Cook Time: 15 minutes

Nutritional Facts/Info:

Calories 781

Carbs 5.9 g

Fat 60.9 g

Protein 50 g

Ingredients:
Hollandaise Sauce
- 2 large egg yolks
- 1 tsp lemon juice
- 2 tbsp butter
- salt and paprika

Eggs Benedict
- 5 oz Canadian bacon, about 4 small slices
- 2 servings 90-second keto mug bread
- 4 large eggs
- salt, as needed
- 1 tbsp white vinegar

- 1 tbsp chives, chopped
- 2 tsp butter

Directions:
1. Prepare the 90-second keto mug bread, slice it into small squares, and place it on the side.
2. Place a pot of water (1–2 inches) to boil on the stove. When the water has boiled, reduce the heat to medium-low and let it simmer.
3. Use a metal bowl to whisk the egg yolks (use a bowl that will fit over the pot).
4. Add the lemon juice and whisk well until incorporated.
5. Melt the butter using a microwave or in a pan over the stove.
6. Once the butter has melted, create a double boiler by placing the bowl over the pot.
7. While the mixture heats up, slowly add in the butter while stirring.
8. Thicken the mixture by stirring continuously. Ensure that the heat is not too high because that will cause the eggs to scramble.
9. You will know that it's ready when the mixture sticks to the back of the spoon, covering it entirely.
10. Sprinkle some salt and pepper on the hollandaise, and allow the flavors to blend for a few minutes.
11. There should be roughly 3–4 inches of water in the pot, so add more if necessary.
12. Bring the water to a boil once more by turning the heat up to medium-high. As soon as it starts to boil, lower the heat and pour in some salt and the vinegar before letting it simmer.
13. The science of the poached egg comes next and, in this step, you need to be extra careful to get that perfect poach, so don't just drop the egg into the water. First,

place the cracked egg into a small dish, then use a spoon or a kebab stick to swirl the water, causing it to spin around the pot as you carefully slide the egg into the center.
14. The egg should take around 2 or 3 minutes depending on how hard or soft you prefer it. Carefully lift the egg out of the water with a slotted spoon before gently touching it to gauge the hardness. Repeat the process with the remaining eggs.
15. Sizzle up the Canadian bacon in a clean pan until lightly browned on both sides, or to your liking.
16. Time to create your eggs Benedict masterpiece by assembling the tower from the slice of mug bread at the bottom, the Canadian bacon, and then the perfect poached egg nestled on top.
17. Complete the dish with a drizzle or a dollop of hollandaise sauce on top, allowing it to ooze down the sides of the egg.
18. Serve, and enjoy!

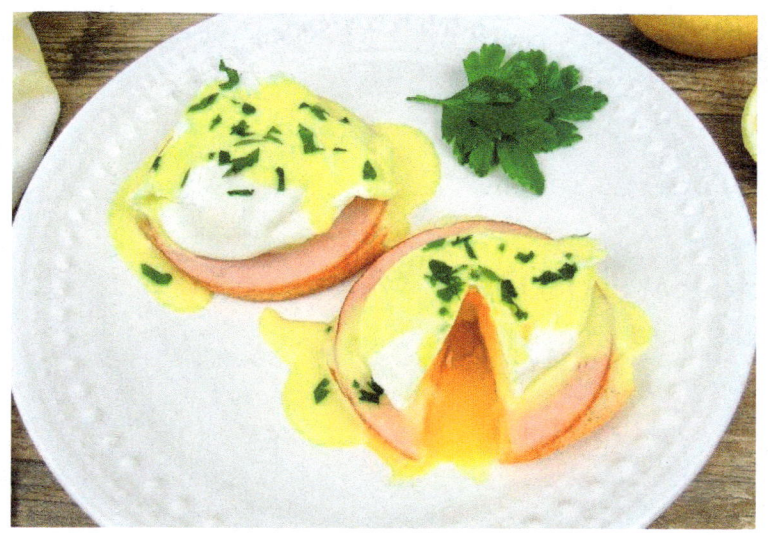

Keto Granola Cereal

Time: 25 minutes
Serving Size: 8 servings

Prep Time: 5 minutes

Cook Time: 20 minutes

Nutritional Facts/Info:

Calories 362

Carbs 4.1 g

Fat 33.5 g

Protein 8.4 g

Ingredients:
- 1 cup almonds
- 1 cup pecans
- 1/2 cup unsweetened shredded coconut
- 1/3 cup sunflower seeds
- 1/3 cup pumpkin seeds
- 1/2 cup golden flaxseed meal
- 6 tbsp erythritol
- 1/2 tsp salt
- 1/2 tsp cinnamon
- 1/4 cup butter, melted
- 1 large egg white
- 1 tsp vanilla extract

Directions:
1. Start by heating the oven to 325°F.
2. Place a sheet of parchment or wax paper over your baking tray.
3. Crumble up the coconut's pieces and almonds, either in a food processor or a blender using the pulse function.
4. Mix in the pecans and repeat the above.
5. Then add the pumpkin seeds, golden flaxseed meal, cinnamon, sunflower seeds, erythritol, and salt and pulse again until everything is combined.
6. Drizzle in the egg white, vanilla extract, and melted butter.
7. Continue with the blending, occasionally using a spoon to scrape up any batter that sticks to the bottom or the sides.
8. Create a thin layer of the granola cereal mixture on the baking sheet, flattening it out where necessary.
9. Allow the granola to bake uninterrupted for approximately 15–18 minutes, watching out for that golden crisp to start forming.
10. Hold off the desire to eat them all up until they cool down, then break them into pieces of whatever size you want.
11. Serve, and enjoy!

Keto Meal Replacement Shake

Time: 5 minutes
Serving Size: 2 servings

Prep Time: 5 minutes

Nutritional Facts/Info:

Calories 453

Carbs 6.9 g

Fat 42.6 g

Protein 8.8 g

Ingredients:
- 1/2 cup heavy cream
- 1/2 medium avocado
- 1 cup unsweetened almond milk, or coconut milk from the carton
- 2 tsp golden flaxseed meal
- 2 tsp almond butter
- 1/2 tsp cinnamon
- 2 tsp cocoa powder
- 1/4 tsp vanilla extract
- 15 drops liquid stevia, or to taste
- 8 whole ice cubes
- 1/8 tsp salt

Directions:
1. Pit and peel the avocado.
2. Add all of your ingredients to a blender, pulse everything together slowly until combined.
3. Blend all the ingredients for 30–45 seconds until a smooth consistency appears.
4. When it comes to the sweetener, add a little and taste to get your desired sweetness.
5. Serve, and enjoy!

Huevos Rancheros

Time: 25 minutes
Serving Size: 1 tostada

Prep Time: 5 minutes

Cook Time: 20 minutes

Nutritional Facts/Info:

Calories 457 | Carbs 6.88 g | Fat 37.33 g | Protein 20.7 g

Ingredients:
Chipotle Salsa
- 2 tbsp coconut oil
- 1/2 medium shallot, finely diced
- 2 tsp crushed red pepper flakes
- 2 tsp minced fresh garlic
- 1/2 cup low-carb tomato sauce, like Rao's
- 2 tsp dried oregano
- salt and pepper, to taste
- 1 tbsp chopped chipotle peppers in adobo sauce

Egg Tortilla
- 2 cups shredded Mexican-style cheese blend
- 1 medium avocado, sliced
- 1/2 medium lime wedges
- 4 large eggs
- 1/4 cup fresh cilantro, chopped

Directions:
1. Melt the coconut oil over medium heat in a skillet.
2. Spoon in the crushed red pepper flakes and allow it to cook until the oil begins to shimmer and the aroma fills the air.
3. Remove the skillet from the stove and set it aside for a few minutes to infuse flavor. Then, strain and discard the solids.
4. Place the skillet on the stove again with some of the drained chili oil. Heat it once more over medium heat.
5. Add the shallots and the onion, then sauté until aromatic.
6. Stir in the allocated amounts of oregano, chipotle chili, and tomato sauce and mix occasionally while watching the sauce reduce slowly as the flavors evaporate off. Turn off the heat and keep the sauce for later.
7. Take out a non-stick pan and, with a paper towel, gently lather the leftover chili oil over the pan, creating a very thin layer.
8. Spread an even layer of cheese on the pan. Cook over low to medium-low heat.
9. When the cheese starts to melt, add the eggs in before covering them with a lid. Give the egg whites time to settle on low heat.
10. As soon as the egg whites begin to firm and the cheese curls up slightly on the side, push up the heat to medium to speed up the cooking time.
11. Consider the "tortilla" done when the bottom layer is uniform and golden-brown.
12. Place the slices of melted cheese and egg tortilla onto a plate.
13. Serve with chili salsa over the top, enjoy!

Keto Breakfast Enchiladas

Time: 55 minutes
Serving Size: ¼ of a casserole

Prep Time: 15 minutes

Cook Time: 40 minutes

Nutritional Facts/Info:

Calories 524.5

Carbs 6.08 g

Fat 42.55 g

Protein 27.3 g

Ingredients:
Tortillas
- ¼ cup heavy whipping cream
- 6 large eggs
- ½ tsp garlic powder
- ½ tsp salt
- ¼ tsp black pepper
- ½ tsp chili powder

Enchiladas
- 8 oz ground sausage
- 1½ cups shredded cheddar cheese
- ¾ cup enchilada sauce

Directions:
1. Preheat a small skillet over a medium-heat stove.
2. Also preheat your oven to 400°F.
3. Use a medium bowl to add the eggs, salt, chili powder, garlic powder, black pepper, and heavy whipping cream.
4. Whisk everything together, and grease the skillet with coconut oil.
5. Drizzle about ¼ cup of the batter into the pan, keeping the heat in with a lid over the top, and allow it to cook all the way through, this should take around 3–5 minutes. Keep repeating this process to get your tortillas.
6. Cook the ground sausage well then set aside.
7. Now be generous when you top each tortilla with spoonfuls of sausage and cheese.
8. Roll them up and place them into a casserole dish.
9. Now pour the enchilada sauce on top, ensuring that you cover all the egg.
10. Sprinkle another layer of cheese over before giving them 15 minutes to bake or until you begin to drool watching the cheese bubble as it melts away.
11. Serve, and enjoy!

Keto Chicken and Waffle Sandwiches

Time: 30 minutes
Serving Size: 4 servings

Prep Time: 15 minutes

Cook Time: 15 minutes

Nutritional Facts/Info:

Calories 452.9

Carbs 5.1 g

Fat 31.68 g

Protein 33.73 g

Ingredients:
Waffles
- 2 tablespoons melted butter
- 1/4 cup milk
- 3 large eggs, yolks, and whites separated
- 1/2 tsp salt
- 1 cup almond flour
- 1 tsp erythritol
- 1 tsp vanilla

Chicken
- 1 cup buttermilk
- 1 large egg

- 2 medium chicken breasts
- oil, for frying
- 1/3 cup almond flour
- 1 tsp paprika
- salt and pepper, to taste
- Optional add-ons: sugar-free syrup, pickles, bacon, and mustard.
- 1/4 tsp cayenne powder

Directions:
1. The night before: Cut the chicken breasts in half lengthwise. Then, once more halve the cut-up pieces lengthwise so you end up with four strips from each breast. Soak the chicken in buttermilk by placing them in a dish in the refrigerator.
2. When you are ready to cook, remove the buttermilk from the dish and season the chicken using salt, pepper, paprika, and cayenne powder.
3. Use a mixing bowl to beat the egg then set the bowl aside.
4. Mix up the almond flour, salt, and pepper in a dry mixing bowl.
5. Create two layers of breading by dipping a chicken strip into the egg and then coating well with almond flour before repeating.
6. In a large skillet, preheat some olive oil. Once the oil is hot flash fry the strips quickly on both sides to crisp up the outer layers.
7. Lay the strips down on a baking sheet and close them up tight by covering them with foil before cooking through in the oven for 15 minutes at 350°F.
8. Preheat your waffle maker.
9. Blend the egg yolks, milk, melted butter, erythritol, and vanilla in a separate bowl by stirring well before

sprinkling in the almond flour and salt and whisking until everything is mixed and consistent.
10. Vigorously mix the egg whites using a hand mixer until it creates mountain-like stiff peaks. Gently fold in half of the peaked egg whites into the prepared batter before folding in the rest.
11. Layer the waffle machine with the oil of your choice before browning 1/3 cup portions of the batter at a time, leaving each portion in for 5–6 minutes or until golden crisp.
12. Place the chicken onto the prepared waffle and add on the optional toppings of your choice.
13. Serve, and enjoy!

Keto Pepperoni Pizza Quiche

Time: 2 hours
Serving Size: 1 quiche

Prep Time: 60 minutes

Cook Time: 60 minutes

Nutritional Facts/Info:

Calories 416.66

Carbs 4.41 g

Fat 38.43 g

Protein 14.29 g

Ingredients:
The Pie Crust:
- 1 ½ cups almond flour
- 1 tsp salt
- ¼ cup coconut flour
- 1 tsp vinegar
- 1 tsp xanthan gum
- 1 large egg, whisked together
- 6 tbsp cold butter, diced

Quiche Filling:
- 1 cup shredded mozzarella cheese
- 6 large eggs

- 15 slices pepperoni
- ½ tsp Italian seasoning
- 1 cup heavy cream
- salt and pepper, to taste
- ¼ tsp red pepper flakes

Directions:
1. Drop the coconut flour, salt, xanthan gum, vinegar, and almond flour into a food processor.
2. Pulse for a little while, before dropping in the butter. Pulse again to create a bread-like consistency.
3. Add the egg to the mixture in the food processor before pulsing some more. This will thicken the dough so it can be rolled into a firm ball before you cover it with plastic and allow it to chill out in the fridge for 45–60 minutes.
4. Preheat the oven to 350°F. Slick a pie plate and piece of foil with a nonstick spray of your choice before setting it aside.
5. Pop the dough onto a piece of parchment paper before covering it with another piece and rolling out a dough circle of roughly 10-inches.
6. Generously pack the pie crust with mozzarella and pepperoni.
7. Use a separate bowl to whisk together the remaining tasty ingredients before drizzling them over the packed pie and add on that extra cheese and pepperoni to top it all off.
8. Bake for 35–45 minutes with a piece of foil covering it to lock in those flavors before removing, giving the pie time to crisp up for another 15 minutes. Check that the eggs have been set before removing them.
9. Serve, and enjoy!

Gooey Keto Cinnamon Rolls

Time: 1 hour
Serving Size: 9 servings

Prep Time: 30 minutes

Cook Time: 30 minutes

Nutritional Facts/Info:

Calories 386.73

Carbs 6.82 g

Fat 31.55 g

Protein 16.62 g

Ingredients:
Cinnamon Rolls
- 1/4 cup sour cream
- 1 tbsps active dry yeast
- 3 tbsps lukewarm water
- 5 tbsps whey protein isolate
- 2 1/4 cups almond flour
- 1 tbsp maple syrup
- 6 tbsps ground golden flaxseed
- 2 1/4 tsp xanthan gum
- 4–6 tbsps erythritol
- Pinch of ground ginger
- 2 1/4 tsp baking powder

- 3 large eggs, room temperature
- 1 1/2 tsp kosher salt
- 1 tbsp apple cider vinegar
- 1 1/2 tbsp unsalted melted butter

Cinnamon Filling
- 2 tbsps ground cinnamon
- 6 tbsps erythritol
- 3 tbsps butter, softened

Glaze
- 3 tbsps unsalted butter
- 1/3 cup cream cheese, room temperature
- 1 tsp vanilla extract
- 3–6 tablespoons powdered erythritol
- heavy cream, as needed
- salt to taste

Directions:
1. Line a baking pan with parchment paper. Smooth out a sheet of cling film over your work space, and keep a bowl with water handy to wet your fingers. You can add a little oil to the water.
2. Add the sour cream, active dry yeast, warm water, and maple syrup in a small bowl and mix.
3. Cover the mixture with a towel and let this sit for 7–10 minutes. The mixture needs to start bubbling to show that the yeast is active.
4. Use a separate bowl to combine the almond flour, whey protein powder, flaxseed meal, xanthan gum, sweetener, baking powder, and salt.
5. Add the eggs, apple cider vinegar, and cooled melted butter to the mixture of yeast. Mix everything with an electric mixture, then add in the flour.

6. Continue mixing until a sticky dough form. Form the dough into a ball with a slightly wet spatula.
7. Now divide the dough into 3 separate dough balls. Spread a small amount of oil on the cling film then add 1 piece of the dough. Wet your fingers (to prevent sticking) and shape them into a rectangle. Coat the dough using the runny butter before sprinkling the cinnamon and erythritol to taste. A 1-inch strip should be left at the top for sealing your roll later.
8. Roll up the dough towards the empty edge using the cling film. Seal the edge of the roll, before using a sharp knife to cut it into 3 equally sized rolls. You will cut easier with a wet knife. Flatten the rolls softly using the palm of your hand before you transfer them to the parchment paper. Repeat this step with the rest of the dough.
9. Use a kitchen towel to cover the pan, then let the dough rise for about an hour. Letting it puff up and double in size.
10. Preheat the oven to 400°F.
11. In the meantime, mix all of the glazing ingredients, use the heavy cream to adjust, if necessary.
12. Bake the rolls until they are a deep golden color. This will take about 20–25 minutes, make sure to remove the tray from the oven after about 10 minutes to cover with tented foil. This helps prevent the rolls from browning too much.
13. Lather on the glaze immediately or while they are steaming as you remove them from the oven.
14. Serve, and enjoy!

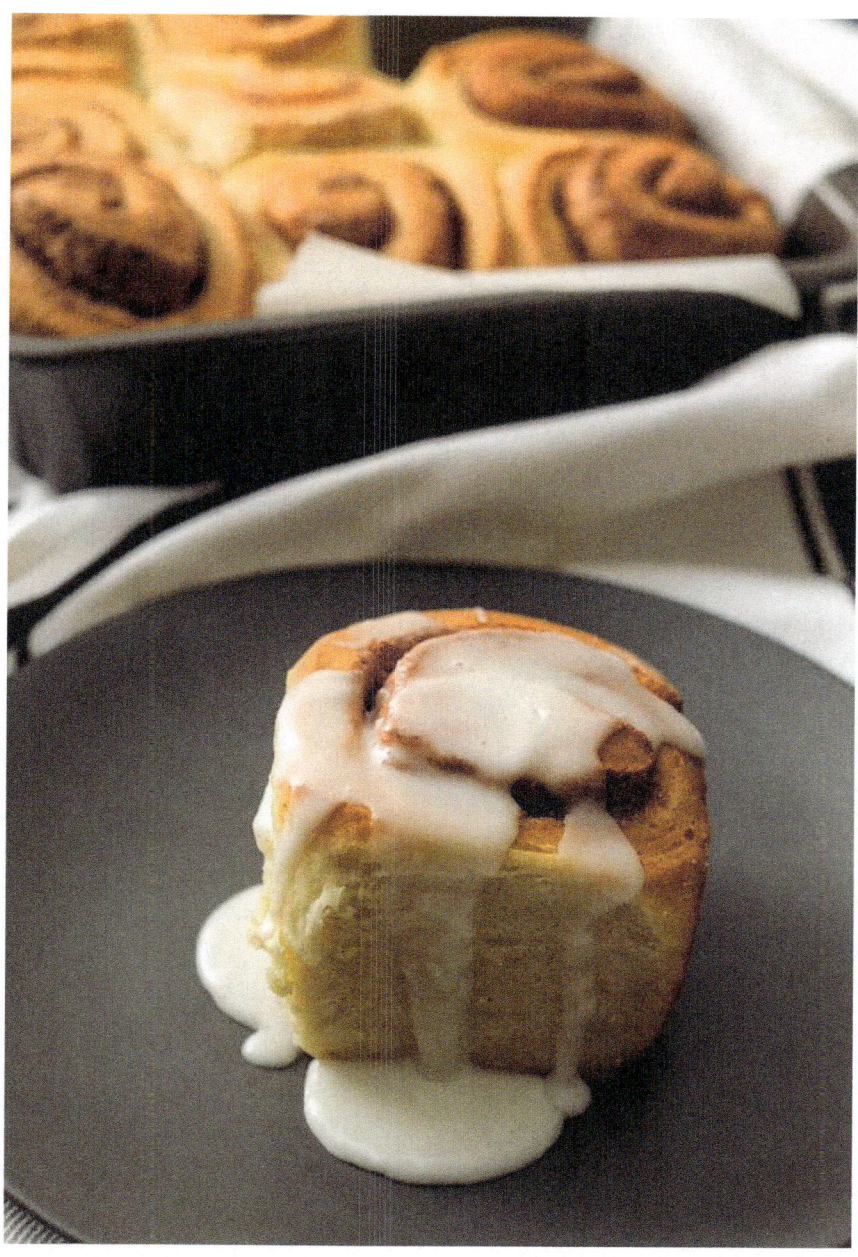

Keto Lemon Sugar Poppy Seed Scones

Time: 40 minutes
Serving Size: 8 servings

Prep Time: 20 minutes

Cook Time: 20 minutes

Nutritional Facts/Info:

Calories 206.81

Carbs 3.53 g

Fat 18.5 g

Protein 6.6 g

Ingredients:
- 1 ½ cups almond flour
- 1 tsp psyllium husk fiber
- 2 tbsps coconut flour
- ¼ tsp baking soda
- 1/2 tsp baking powder
- 4 tbsps butter
- 1 tbsp poppy seeds
- 2 large eggs
- ¼ cup erythritol
- 2 tbsp erythritol, for sprinkling
- ½ lemon, juice, and zest

Directions:
1. First, preheat the oven to 350°F.
2. Then line a baking sheet with parchment paper.
3. Use a large mixing bowl to combine almond flour, coconut flour, baking powder, psyllium husk fiber, and baking soda. Add in poppy seeds until well combined.
4. Now, add the cut butter in with the dry ingredients using a fork, or your hands to create a dough.
5. Use a separate bowl to whisk together the eggs and sweeteners until they are frothy.
6. Zest lemon onto a plate, then adds the sprinkling erythritol. Use a fork to meld the sugar and zest together and place it on the side to dry.
7. Slice the lemon in half before squeezing the juice into the egg mixture, remove any lemon seeds that fall into the mix.
8. Add the egg mixture into the dough and mix well then place the wet dough onto the parchment shaped into a dome.
9. Score the dough in 8 triangles with a knife and pop in the oven to bake for 20 minutes.
10. Take them out of the oven and cut them into 8 triangles before separating each slice. Sprinkle some lemon sugar before baking for another 10 minutes.
11. Serve, and enjoy!

Bacon Kale and Tomato Frittata

Time: 20 minutes
Serving Size: 6 servings

Prep Time: 10 minutes

Cook Time: 10 minutes

Nutritional Facts/Info:

Calories 292.5

Carbs 1.61 g

Fat 24.88 g

Protein 13.77 g

Ingredients:
- 7 strips bacon
- 1 cup (2 ounces) chopped kale, stems removed
- 7 large eggs
- ¼ cup heavy whipping cream
- 1 tbsp mayonnaise
- ½ cup shredded Parmesan cheese
- 2 sprigs parsley, chopped, to garnish
- 5 cherry tomatoes, sliced

Directions:
1. Heat oven to 400°F.
2. Use a large bowl to beat the eggs, mayonnaise, and heavy whipping cream until combined. Then add Parmesan cheese, mix gently, and put to the side.
3. Place a non-stick skillet over medium-low heat and sauté the bacon until crisp. Once crisp, place bacon on a paper towel to cool and drain the excess grease. Keep one strip for garnish.
4. Use the skillet you fried the bacon in, and lightly fry kale using medium or low heat until the leaves are wilting and soft.
5. Crumble the bacon into the skillet and mix up the greens and meat evenly.
6. Stir the egg mixture to ensure that any cheese that has settled at the bottom is incorporated.
7. Now pour the egg mixture into the skillet over medium heat.
8. Watch the eggs carefully and add 3/4 of the tomato halves as the eggs start to set and cook for a further minute.
9. Just as the frittata starts setting around the edges, place the skillet in the oven for about 5–10 minutes.
10. Serve, and enjoy!

Vegan Keto Scramble

Time: 15 minutes
Serving Size: 5 servings

Prep Time: 10 minutes

Cook Time: 5 minutes

Nutritional Facts/Info:

Calories 211.4

Carbs 4.74 g

Fat 17.56 g

Protein 10.09 g

Ingredients:
- 3 tbsp avocado oil
- 1 14-oz package firm tofu
- 1 1/2 tsp nutritional yeast
- 2 tbsps diced yellow onion
- 1/2 tsp turmeric
- 1/2 tsp garlic powder
- 1 cup baby spinach
- 1/2 tsp salt
- 3 oz vegan cheddar cheese
- 3 grape tomatoes

Directions:
1. First, press the tofu block by covering it with a few layers of paper towel, and place something heavy on it to remove excess water. Then set it aside.
2. Place a skillet on medium heat, and fry the chopped onion in 1/3 of the avocado oil, when it is sizzling translucent, it is ready.
3. Add the block of tofu into the skillet and crumble it using a fork until it resembles the consistency of a scrambled egg.
4. Coat the tofu by drizzling the rest of the oil before sprinkling over the dry seasoning.
5. Continue cooking over medium heat, stirring occasionally to let most of the liquid evaporate.
6. Now add in the baby spinach, diced tomato, and cheese for one minute. You will know it's ready when the spinach has wilted and the cheese has melted.
7. Serve hot, and enjoy!

Keto Sausage Gravy and Biscuit Bake

Time: 40 minutes
Serving Size: 6 servings

Prep Time: 10 minutes

Cook Time: 30 minutes

Nutritional Facts/Info:

Calories 374.67

Carbs 4.75 g

Fat 33.21 g

Protein 14.48 g

Ingredients:
Biscuits:
- 1 cup almond flour
- ½ tsp xanthan gum
- 1 tsp baking powder
- 2 egg whites
- 2 tbsps butter, frozen

Sausage gravy:
- 12 oz ground pork breakfast sausage
- 1 ½ cups chicken broth
- 1 tsp xanthan gum
- 1 tsp black pepper

- ½ tsp onion powder
- ½ cup half and half
- ¼ tsp salt, to taste

Directions:
1. Use a large bowl to mix the almond flour, ½ tsp xanthan gum, and baking powder.
2. Grate the butter while it is still frozen. Then add it into the mixture of flour and mix with a fork until it creates coarse crumbs. Set it aside.
3. Use a separate medium-size bowl and create stiff peaks by beating the white of the eggs.
4. Fold the egg whites into the flour crumbs mixture with a rubber spatula until just combined.
5. Place the biscuit mixture in the refrigerator to chill while you make the gravy.
6. In a large skillet, fry the sausage over medium heat till it is browned.
7. Remove the sausage and place it on a paper towel-lined plate to drain the excess oil, leave a tablespoon of fat in the skillet.
8. Re-adjust the heat to a medium temperature then pour 1 tsp of xanthan gum into the grease, while constantly mixing. The xanthan gum should take about a minute before it begins to brown.
9. Add and mix in the onion powder, chicken stock, and black pepper.
10. Let the mix simmer away slowly bubbling and thickening to a creamy sauce for around 5 minutes.
11. Keep it simmering away while you stir in the half and half, creating a thick and creamy gravy.
12. Add in the sausage and coat it evenly with the gravy before you take it off the heat.
13. Preheat the oven to 375°F.

14. Transfer the sausage gravy into an 8" x 8" inch casserole dish.
15. Dust the top of the gravy with the biscuit in small amounts until a thick layer is formed, be sure to evenly distribute it on the gravy.
16. Bake for 20 minutes until it starts to bubble and you can smell the warm flavors steaming off the biscuits which should be slightly browned.
17. Serve, and enjoy!

No-potatoes Bubble and Squeak

Time: 40 minutes
Serving Size: 3 servings

Prep Time: 10 minutes

Cook Time: 30 minutes

Nutritional Facts/Info:

Calories 332.67

Carbs 8.6 g

Fat 28.11 g

Protein 10.65 g

Ingredients:
Mashed Cauliflower
- ½ medium cauliflower, cut into florets
- salt and pepper to taste
- 2 tbsps heavy whipping cream
- 1 tbsp butter

Bubble n Squeak
- 3 slices bacon, diced
- 50 g leek, sliced
- 1 tbsp butter
- ¼ medium onion, diced
- 50 g chopped Brussels sprouts

- 1 stalk green onion, sliced
- ¼ cup grated Parmesan
- ¼ cup grated mozzarella
- 1 tsp minced garlic
- 2 tbsp duck fat

Directions:
1. You can use some leftover mashed cauliflower for this recipe. If you do not have this use the cauliflower florets and place in a medium-size bowl with 1 tablespoon of butter and cream. Microwave on high for 4 minutes uncovered. Stir to prevent the cauliflower from drying.
2. Then pop it back in for another 4 minutes.
3. Blend the cauliflower until creamy in an immersion blender. Expect it to be considerably thick. Now add the mozzarella to melt while still hot. And set this aside to cool.
4. Crisp up the topped bacon until sizzling and fragrant in a hot pan with a small amount of oil.
5. Then remove the bacon and place it on a paper towel.
6. Melt 1 tbsp of butter in the remaining bacon fat before tossing in the garlic until fragrant and soft, this should take about a minute.
7. Introduce the onion and fry it for around 3–5 minutes, or until the onion is soft and translucent.
8. Add and cook down the Brussels sprouts and roughly chopped leeks in the mixture for 5–10 minutes.
9. Now add the green onions to the pan and cook quickly for only 1 minute. Do not cook for too long so that the green onions reserve some of their freshness.
10. Turn off the stove and leave the contents of the pan to cool down.

11. Drop the bacon into the vegetable mixture, before stirring it all into the mashed cauliflower.
12. Once the flavors have melded, warm up the empty pan on medium to high heat before tossing in the duck fat. Place the egg rings into the melted fat before throwing in some parmesan inside the rings.
13. Now add the cauliflower mix into the rings and sprinkle Parmesan again on top this time.
14. Turnover and allow to cook until a crispy crust form.
15. Serve, and enjoy!

Lemon Raspberry Sweet Rolls

Time: 40 minutes
Serving Size: 8 servings

Prep Time: 10 minutes

Cook Time: 30 minutes

Nutritional Facts/Info:

Calories 272.25

Carbs 5.24 g

Fat 23.18 g

Protein 10.04 g

Ingredients:
For the lemon cream cheese filling:
- 2 tbsp stevia erythritol blend*
- 2 tbsp butter, room temperature
- 4 oz cream cheese, room temperature
- 1 tsp lemon extract
- ½ tsp vanilla extract
- 1 tsp lemon juice
- Zest from one lemon (about 2 teaspoons)

For the raspberry sauce:
- 1 tbsp water
- ¼ tbsp xanthan gum

- 2 tbsps stevia erythritol blend
- ½ cup frozen raspberries
- 2 tsp lemon juice

For the dough:
- ¼ tsp xanthan gum
- ¼ cup stevia erythritol blend
- 1 cup superfine almond flour
- 1 large egg
- 1 ¼ tsp baking powder
- 2 cups part-skim mozzarella cheese
- 1 tsp vanilla extract

For the lemon glaze: (optional)
- ¼ tsp vanilla extract
- ½ ounce cream cheese, room temperature
- 2 tbsps butter, room temperature
- 1 tsp lemon juice
- 2 tbsps stevia erythritol blend
- 1 ½ tbsps unsweetened almond milk, room temperature
- ¼ tsp lemon extract

Directions:
1. With an electric mixer beat the cream cheese, vanilla extract, lemon extract, butter, sweetener, lemon zest, and lemon juice to create a consistently smooth paste. Leave it for later.

Raspberry Sauce:
2. Use a medium saucepan to whisk the sweetener and xanthan gum together. Then gradually add water and lemon juice while whisking.

3. Set heat to medium-low then add frozen raspberries, making sure that you stir constantly. When the sauce begins to simmer, remove from heat, and place it aside.

Dough:
4. Preheat the oven to 350°F. Then grease a 9" circular pan with the fat of your choice. Have your two 15-inch sheets of parchment and a rolling pin ready for action a little later.
5. Prepare your double boiler. A medium saucepan with a medium bowl that will sit on top can also work in this instance.
6. Add 2 inches of water to the saucepan. Place the saucepan over high heat and wait for it to simmer uncovered. As the simmering begins, drop the heat down low.
7. Meanwhile in the top part of the double boiler combine the almond flour, xanthan gum, stevia/erythritol sweetener, and baking powder using a whisk or fork.
8. Then stir in the egg and vanilla extract. The mixture should look very thick.
9. Fold in the mozzarella cheese and put the bowl over the pot of simmering water.
10. Keep stirring the mixture constantly, the cheese will melt and combine with the flour. It should look like bread dough.
11. Once the cheese has melted completely, take out the dough and put it on a piece of parchment paper that has been pre-prepared. Knead the dough a bit to completely combine the flour mixture and the cheese. Shape the dough into a rectangular shape and cover it with the other piece of parchment. Roll out dough creating 12" x 15" rectangles. Then remove the top parchment.

12. Lather the lemon cream cheese filling covering the dough, while leaving about ½ inch uncovered on the edges. And top it off by spooning the raspberry sauce over the lemon cream cheese filling and spreading it evenly.
13. Begin at the longer side and start to roll the dough into a log shape and press the outside long edge to seal.
14. Using a serrated knife, gently cut the log crosswise into 8 pieces. Place one roll in the center of the prepared pan and the rest circled it.
15. Bake for 24 minutes or until the tops look smooth and golden brown.

Lemon glaze:
16. Use a small bowl to beat cream cheese and butter with an electric mixer until smooth.
17. Add vanilla, lemon juice, sweetener, and lemon extract and blend until combined.
18. Slowly add the almond milk, about a teaspoon at a time, vigorously beating the mix each time.
19. Serve, and enjoy!

Blueberry Ricotta Pancakes

Time: 20 minutes
Serving Size: 5 servings

Prep Time: 10 minutes

Cook Time: 10 minutes

Nutritional Facts/Info:

Calories 311.4

Carbs 5.78 g

Fat 22.61 g

Protein 15.25 g

Ingredients:
- 3 large eggs
- ¾ cup ricotta
- ¼ cup unsweetened vanilla almond milk
- ½ tsp vanilla extract
- ½ cup golden flaxseed meal
- 1 cup almond flour
- 1 tsp baking powder
- ¼ tsp salt
- ¼ cup blueberries
- ¼–½ tsp stevia powder

Directions:
1. Preheat a skillet over medium heat.
2. Blend the eggs, ricotta, vanilla extract, and unsweetened almond milk.
3. Then mix the almond flour, salt, golden flaxseed meal, stevia, and baking powder in a separate bowl.
4. Now slowly add all of the dry ingredients into the blender, and blend until a smooth consistency of batter forms.
5. Of ¼ cup of blueberries, you will need to add 3 blueberries per pancake (or as desired).
6. Add butter to the preheated skillet. Then let the butter melt.
7. Drizzle your pancake batter into the skillet and flip your pancake when lightly browned on the outside.
8. Serve with sugar-free syrup or additional berries.

Keto Lemon Poppyseed Muffins

Time: 30 minutes
Serving Size: 12 servings

Prep Time: 10 minutes

Cook Time: 20 minutes

Nutritional Facts/Info:

Calories 99.89

Carbs 1.73 g

Fat 11.69 g

Protein 4.04 g

Ingredients:
- ¼ cup golden flaxseed meal
- ¾ cup almond flour
- 1 tsp baking powder
- 1/3 cup erythritol
- ¼ cup salted butter, melted
- 2 tbsps poppy seeds
- 3 large eggs
- ¼ cup heavy cream
- 3 tbsps lemon juice
- zest of 2 lemons
- 25 drops liquid stevia
- 1 tsp vanilla extract

Directions:
1. Preheat the oven to 350°F.
2. Use a bowl to combine almond flour, erythritol, flaxseed meal, and poppy seeds and mix.
3. Now stir in the eggs, melted butter, and heavy cream until smooth.
4. Then add the baking powder, lemon zest, vanilla, stevia, and lemon juice. Mix again until the ingredients are all incorporated.
5. Pour the batter out equally between 12 cupcake molds.
6. Bake for 20 minutes or until slight browning appears.
7. Take them out of the oven and hold off the hunger pains for about 10 minutes so that they can cool down and the flavors can develop.
8. Slice and serve!

Chapter 4: Recipes for Lunch

Keto Lunch Recipes

Ham and Cheese Keto Stromboli

Time: 50 minutes
Serving Size: 2 servings

Prep Time: 15 minutes

Cook Time: 20–25 minutes

Nutritional Facts/Info:

Calories 350 | Carbs 3.7 g | Fat 25.2 g | Protein 26.8 g

Ingredients:
- 4 oz of ham
- 3 1/2 oz cheddar cheese
- 4 tbsps of almond flour
- 1 1/4 cups of shredded mozzarella cheese
- 1 large egg
- 3 tbsps of coconut flour
- 1 tsp of Italian seasoning
- pepper
- salt

Directions:
1. Let the oven reach a high of 400°F and use your microwave to melt the mozzarella cheese. This should take 1 minute. Be careful not to overheat the cheese. Stir occasionally to ensure that the entire cheese has melted.
2. Mix your almond and coconut flour together, as well as the seasonings in a mixing bowl. You can use seasonings of your choice; I used Italian seasoning, pepper, and salt.
3. Once the mozzarella has melted, pour it into your flour mixture to work it in nicely.
4. After about 1 minute, the cheese will have had time to cool a bit, then add in your egg and mix everything.
5. When everything is mixed, you will have a moist dough, settle it on some parchment paper laid out on a flat surface.
6. Cover the ball of dough using another piece of parchment paper and with a rolling pin or your hand flatten it out.
7. Cut diagonal lines from the edge of the dough to the center using a knife or a pizza cutter, then leave a row of your dough untouched about 4-inches wide.
8. Alternate laying the ham and then, the cheddar on the uncut stretch of dough.
9. Lift one section of your dough at a time and lay it over the top, to encase the yummy smelling filling.
10. Bake for approximately 15 to 20 minutes till it has turned golden brown.
11. Serve and enjoy!

Prosciutto, Caramelized Onion, & Parmesan Braid

Time: 50 minutes
Serving Size: 4 servings

Prep Time: 10 minutes

Cook Time: 40 minutes

Nutritional Facts/Info:

Calories 198

Carbs 5 g

Fat 14.4 g

Protein 12.5 g

Ingredients:
- 1 tbsp of butter
- 1 egg
- 3 oz of prosciutto (sliced thinly)
- 1 medium onion (finely chopped)
- 2 cups of part-skim mozzarella cheese (finely grated)
- 1 tsp of balsamic vinegar
- 2 tsp of minced fresh basil
- 1 clove of crushed garlic
- 3/4 cup of almond flour
- 1/2 cup + 1 tbsp of finely grated Parmesan cheese
- 1/2 tsp of salt

- freshly ground black pepper
- olive oil (optional)

Directions:
1. Warm up the oven to a toasty 375°F. Prepare 2 pieces of parchment on the side, a rolling pin, and a baking sheet.
2. Place a large-sized skillet over a medium heat stove, then add the butter. Allow the butter to melt till it starts foaming, then add your onions. Cook the onions, stirring occasionally until the edges brown and the onions begin to caramelize.
3. Now add your garlic to your skillet. Cook for 1 minute, stirring constantly. Pour the balsamic vinegar over the caramelized onions and cook until almost completely evaporated.
4. Add your prosciutto to your skillet, separating the thin slices before laying them in your skillet. Cook them while stirring for about 1 minute. Now, add in your basil, then remove your skillet from the heat. Taste and adjust seasoning with salt and pepper.
5. Prepare a double boiler and bring your water in the lower part of your double boiler to a simmer. The top part of your double boiler should hold the almond flour, mozzarella cheese, and salt.
6. Take the top part of the boiler containing the almond flour and mozzarella mixture over the bottom part with your simmering water. Heat your mixture, while constantly stirring, until the cheese melts and the mixture becomes a dough-like ball. Be careful not to burn yourself with the steam coming from the boiler.
7. Take your mozzarella dough and place it onto a piece of parchment paper. Knead it several times to make sure that any stray almond flour is incorporated into

your dough and completely mix your cheese and your almond flour. Pat your dough into an oval shape. Cover your dough with a second piece of parchment and spread it out into an oblong shape about 14" x 9"-inches using a roller.

8. Now, spread the filling along with the middle third of the dough, making sure to leave about 1/3 of the dough on both sides. Then sprinkle 1/2 cup of your Parmesan cheese over your filling.
9. Cut about 1-inch wide strips down the sides to where your filling starts. Crisscross the strips to ensure that there is an equal number on either side but be careful towards the end as you should be able to fold the bottom over the filling and cross the last few strips over top.
10. Break your egg into your small-sized bowl. Whisk lightly and brush over your bread. Sprinkle your loaf with your reserved Parmesan cheese and sprinkle as much black pepper as you desire.
11. Bake in your preheated oven for 18 to 22 minutes or until it is golden brown. While smelling the flavors wafting around the room, hold in your desire to devour it for 5 minutes as it cools on the baking sheet, before placing it on a cutting board.
12. Slice, serve, and enjoy!

Spaghetti Squash with Meatballs

Time: 1hour 30 minutes
Serving Size: 4 servings

Prep Time: 30 minutes

Cook Time: 1 hour

Nutritional Facts/Info:

Calories 1448

Carbs 56.2 g

Fat 80.2 g

Protein 131.1 g

Ingredients:
Beef Meatballs:
- 16 oz of ground beef (80/20)
- 1/3 onion
- 1/3 green pepper
- 1 egg
- 1 tbsp of minced garlic
- 2 oz of shredded cheddar cheese
- 1 tbsp of coconut flour
- salt
- pepper

Pork Meatballs:

- 16 oz of ground pork
- 1 egg
- 1/3 green pepper
- 2 oz of shredded Monterey Jack cheese
- 1/3 onion
- 1 tbsp of almond flour
- 1 tbsp of minced garlic
- salt
- pepper

Chicken Meatballs:
- 16 oz of ground chicken thighs
- 1/3 green pepper
- 1 egg
- 1/3 onion
- 1 tbsp of minced garlic
- 2 oz of shredded Jarlsberg cheese
- 1 tbsp of ground flax meal
- salt
- pepper

Spaghetti:
- 2 1/4 lbs of spaghetti squash (cooked and shredded)
- 10 tsp of Parmesan cheese
- 24 oz of Rao's Homemade Marinara Sauce

Directions:
1. Cut the spaghetti squash in two halves and scrape out the insides.
2. Place it face down in your glass container and add some water until it rises above your cut portion.
3. Cook for approximately 45 minutes at 375°F.
4. Dice the onions and pepper then divide up into three separate parts.

5. Now combine the beef, 1/3 of your onions and peppers, 1 egg, cheddar cheese, coconut flour, pepper, salt, and garlic.
6. Use your hands to divide this up into 10 separate meatballs. They should be about 1 1/2 oz each.
7. Then place them on your baking sheet that's been lined with foil.
8. Combine the pork, 1/3 of your onions and peppers, 1 egg, almond flour, pepper, salt, garlic, and Monterey Jack cheese.
9. Use your hands to divide this up into 10 separate meatballs.
10. Place them on your baking sheet that's been lined with foil.
11. Combine your pork, 1/3 of your onions and peppers, 1 egg, ground flax meal, pepper, salt, garlic, and Jarlsberg cheese.
12. Use your hands to divide this up into 10 separate meatballs. Should be about 1 ½ oz each.
13. Place them on your baking sheet that's been lined with foil.
14. Cook them at 375°F for approximately 25 minutes.
15. Place 1/10 of your spaghetti squash, 1 of each type of meatball, 2 ounces of marinara, and 1 oz of shredded Parmesan cheese into each container. You'll need 10 containers in total.
16. Serve, and enjoy!

Easy Shrimp Avocado Salad with Tomatoes

Time: 20 min
Serving Size: 2 servings

Prep Time: 10 min

Cook Time: 2 min

Nutritional Facts/Info:

Calories 529

Carbs 16.9 g

Fat 13 g

Protein 28.8 g

Ingredients:
- 1 handful cherry tomatoes, diced
- 1 large avocado, diced
- 8 oz (225 g) raw shrimp, peeled and deveined
- freshly chopped cilantro (or parsley)
- 1/2 red onion, minced
- 1 tbsp lime juice
- 2 tbsps salted butter, melted
- salt and fresh cracked pepper
- 1 tbsp olive oil

Directions:
1. The shrimp avocado salad preparation: Toss shrimp and melted butter into a bowl and flip the shrimp around until well-coated.
2. Heat a skillet over medium to high heat. Then add some shrimp to the skillet, leave them in for about a minute or until they look pink around the edges. Now flip them over to another side and cook until shrimp are cooked through. This should take less than a minute.
3. Transfer shrimp to a plate to allow them to cool while you get busy with the other ingredients.
4. Add all other ingredients (avocado, tomatoes, parsley, and red onion) into a large mixing bowl. Sprinkle them with some olive oil and lime juice and toss them around to mix everything.
5. Now add the cooked shrimp and give a quick stir to mix everything. Season the shrimp avocado salad with salt and pepper, to taste.
6. Serve and enjoy!

Baked Greek Chicken with Feta & Dill

Time: 40 minutes
Serving Size: 4 servings

Prep Time: 5 minutes

Cook Time: 35 minutes

Nutritional Facts/Info:

Calories 393

Carbs 4 g

Fat 18 g

Protein 50 g

Ingredients:
- 2 lb frozen chicken tenders
- 1/2-pint tomatoes
- 2 tbsp avocado oil
- 1 large zucchini
- 1/2 tsp salt
- 3 sprigs fresh dill
- 1 tbsp fresh dill finely chopped
- 1 tbsp lemon juice
- 2 tbsp feta cheese, finely chopped
- 1 tbsp extra virgin olive oil

Directions:
1. Preheat the oven to 400°F.
2. Drizzle the avocado oil on a large sheet pan (you can use any other vegetable oil of your choice). Then, place the chicken, dill, tomatoes, and zucchini on the tray. Season with salt and bake for about 30 minutes.
3. In the meantime, take the toppings (the dill, feta, lemon juice, and olive oil) and stir them together.
4. The chicken should be ready after 30 minutes in the oven. Take the chicken out of the oven and place it on a serving tray. Then bake the vegetables in the oven for 3–5 minutes until they look brown and roasted. Then you can discard the cooked dill sprigs.
5. Now, put the vegetables over the chicken on the serving tray. Sprinkle the feta mixture on top.
6. Serve, and enjoy!

Air Fryer Turkey Meatballs

Time: 15 mins
Serving Size: 4 servings

Prep Time: 5 mins

Cook Time: 10 min

Nutritional Facts/Info:

Calories 220

Carbs 2 g

Fat 4 g

Protein 42 g

Ingredients:
- 1.5 lb (675 g) turkey mince
- 1 red bell pepper, deseeded and finely chopped
- 1 large egg, lightly beaten
- 4 tbsps minced fresh herbs parsley
- 1 tbsp minced fresh cilantro coriander
- salt
- black pepper
- cooking spray

Directions:
1. Preheat the air fryer to 400°F.
2. Mix all the ingredients (leaving out the cooking spray) together in a large bowl.
3. Use your hands to shape the mixture into 4-inch meatballs.
4. Place half of the meatballs in a single-layer air fryer basket.
5. Cook for 7–10 mins until they are lightly browned and cooked through. (Shake the meatballs at about 4 minutes in to give them a turn).
6. Remove them from the fryer and keep warm, and repeat with the remaining meatball mixture.
7. Serve them warm with any side of your choice or deep sauce, and enjoy!

Cucumber Tomato Salad

Time: 10 mins
Serving Size: 6 servings

Prep Time: 10 mins

Nutritional Facts/Info:

Calories 62

Carbs 4 g

Fat 4 g

Protein 0 g

Ingredients:
For the salad:
- 375 g cherry tomatoes grape tomatoes, halved
- 1 cucumber deseeded and cubed
- 3 tbsp red onion chopped
- 2 tbsp fresh dill chopped
- 1 tsp dried oregano

For the dressing:
- 2 tbsp apple cider vinegar
- 2 tbsp extra virgin olive oil
- pinch of salt

Directions:

For the salad:
1. Add cherry tomatoes, red onion, cucumber, oregano, and dill to a large bowl and mix to combine.

For the dressing:
1. Pour the olive oil and apple cider vinegar into a jar or small bottle, add a pinch of salt and shake till everything is well incorporated.
2. Drizzle the dressing on top of the salad.
3. Serve, and enjoy!

Cheddar Broccoli Soup

Time: 35 minutes
Serving Size: 4 servings

Prep Time: 10 minutes

Cook Time: 25 minutes

Nutritional Facts/Info:

Calories 282

Carbs 9.5 g

Fat 19 g

Protein 19.5 g

Ingredients:
- 1/2 white onion
- 1 cup of heavy cream
- 1 tbsp of butter
- 8 oz of cheddar
- 2 cups of broth
- 12 ounces of broccoli
- 2 cups of water
- 1/4 tsp of xanthan gum
- 1/2 tsp of paprika
- salt
- pepper

Directions:
1. Place a large-sized pot on medium heat, then add a tablespoon of butter.
2. Add garlic and onion to the pot of butter to sauté till the onion looks translucent.
3. Add the broth, cream, and water. Then allow everything to come to a boil. Season with your salt, pepper, and paprika.
4. While boiling, rip the broccoli into pieces of florets and measure 12 ounces. Then, place them into the boiling soup broth and reduce the heat to a simmer. Allow the broccoli to cook for approximately 25 minutes.
5. Once your broccoli is cooked, add 8 ounces of cheddar cheese and stir it in until melted. Shredded cheese will melt faster than cubed cheese.
6. After your cheese has melted, turn off the heat. Pour the soup into a large-sized blender and continue to blend until everything is smooth. An immersion blender would work perfectly fine as well.
7. When blending, slowly add in a 1/4 teaspoon of your xanthan gum. Then, you should notice your soup thickening.
8. When finished, sprinkle some cheddar cheese on top.
9. Serve and enjoy

Avocado Tuna Melt Bites

Time: 20 min
Serving Size: 12 servings

Prep Time: 10 minutes

Cook Time: 10 minutes

Nutritional Facts/Info:

Calories 197

Carbs 3.4 g

Fat 17.5 g

Protein 7.5 g

Ingredients:
- 10 oz of canned tuna (drained)
- 1/3 cup of almond flour
- 1/4 cup of mayonnaise
- 1/4 cup of parmesan cheese
- 1 medium avocado (cubed)
- 1/2 tsp of garlic powder
- 1/2 cup of coconut oil
- 1/4 tsp of onion powder
- pepper
- salt

Directions:
1. Drain your can of tuna and add it to a large-sized bowl which you will use to mix everything.
2. Now, add some mayonnaise, Parmesan cheese, and spices to your tuna and mix everything.
3. Slice your avocado in half and cube the insides.
4. Now, add the cubed avocado into your tuna mixture and fold together, being careful not to mash the avocado in the process.
5. Form your tuna mixture into balls and roll in your almond flour, covering completely. Then put the balls aside on a tray or in a wide dish.
6. Heat your coconut oil in a pan over medium heat. When the pan is hot enough, add the tuna balls and fry them till they are crisp on both sides.
7. Remove from your pan.
8. Serve warm, and enjoy

Homemade Keto Caesar Salad

Time: 30 minutes
Serving Size: 2 servings

Prep Time: 10 minutes

Cook Time: 20 minutes

Nutritional Facts/Info:

Calories 997

Carbs 4.9 g

Fat 74.35 g

Protein 71.75 g

Ingredients:
Salad
- salt and pepper, to taste
- 1 tbsp olive oil
- 10 oz boneless, skinless chicken breast
- 8 oz romaine lettuce
- 2 oz cooked bacon
- 1 oz Parmesan cheese, grated

Dressing
- 1/2 medium lemon, zest, and juice
- 1 tbsp Dijon mustard
- 1/2 cup mayonnaise

- 2 tbsp finely chopped anchovy fillets
- 1/2 oz Parmesan cheese, grated
- salt and pepper, to taste
- 1 tsp minced garlic

Directions:
1. Preheat the oven to 350°F.
2. Mix all of the dressing ingredients and blend or whisk together until combined. Then set it aside in the refrigerator.
3. Now put the chicken breasts into a baking dish and drizzle olive oil over the chicken, making sure that the oil coats the top and the bottom.
4. Season with salt and pepper to your liking, and cook in the oven for roughly 20 minutes or until chicken is fully cooked through.
5. Assemble the salad with lettuce, chicken, bacon, and all the dressing ingredients mixed. Finish it off with a sprinkle of the grated parmesan cheese.
6. Serve, and enjoy!

Grilled Tuna Salad with Garlic Dressing

Time: 25 minutes
Serving Size: 2 servings

Prep Time: 10 minutes

Cook Time: 15 minutes

Nutritional Facts/Info:

Calories 743

Carbs 9.8 g

Fat 58.4 g

Protein 40.9 g

Ingredients:
- 1 tbsp olive oil
- 8 oz asparagus spears
- 2 large eggs
- 4 oz spring mix
- 8 oz fresh tuna
- 1/2 medium red onion
- 2 oz cherry tomatoes
- 1/2 cup mayonnaise
- 2 tbsps walnuts, chopped
- 2 tsp garlic powder
- 2 tbsps water
- salt and pepper to taste

Directions:
1. Use a bowl to put together the mayonnaise, water, garlic powder, and salt and pepper creating a delicious creamy dressing.
2. Stir the mixture well until combined and put it aside.
3. Boil the eggs for about 8–10 minutes. Then allow them to cool, then peel and slice them in half.
4. Now, wash and cut the asparagus into equal lengths. Then fry the asparagus separately in a pan.
5. Rub the olive oil onto both sides of the fresh tuna equally and fry for 3–5 minutes on each side. Season the tuna with salt and pepper, according to your preference.
6. Arrange the greens, cherry tomato halves, onion, and eggs on a plate.
7. Slice the grilled tuna into strips and place it on top.
8. Cover the salad with a drizzle of creamy dressing and sprinkle the chopped walnuts on top.

Keto Cloud Bread BLT

Time: 40 minutes
Serving Size: 1 sandwich

Prep Time: 20 minutes

Cook Time: 20 minutes

Nutritional Facts/Info:

Calories 527.93

Carbs 4.83 g

Fat 46.98 g

Protein 19.75 g

Ingredients:
Cloud bread
- 3 large eggs
- 4¼ oz softened cream cheese
- salt, to taste
- ½ tbsp ground psyllium husk powder
- ½ tsp baking powder
- ¼ tsp cream of tartar

Toppings
- 8 tbsps mayonnaise
- 5 oz bacon, cooked
- 2 oz lettuce

- 1 large tomato, thinly sliced

Directions:
1. Preheat your oven to 300°F.
2. Separate the eggs into whites and yolks.
3. Add some salt and cream of tartar to the egg whites and whip until very stiff with a hand mixer.
4. Mix the cream cheese, psyllium husk powder, and egg yolks.
5. Gently fold the egg whites into the runny egg yolks. Be careful not to overmix and cause the egg whites to lose their whip.
6. Place some parchment paper on a baking sheet. Shape the batter into 8 rounds then bake for 25 minutes, or until golden.
7. Turn the cloud bread pieces over so their tops face down. Spread 1 tablespoon across each.
8. Stack the bacon, lettuce, and tomato on top of four of the bread pieces.
9. Serve, and enjoy!

Ketofied Chick-Fil-A-Style Chicken

Time: 40 minutes
Serving Size: 2 servings

Prep Time: 10 minutes

Cook Time: 30 minutes

Nutritional Facts/Info:

Calories 342.53

Carbs 1.68 g

Fat 14.8 g

Protein 47.6 g

Ingredients:
- 2 scoops unflavored 100% whey protein powder
- 8 medium uncooked chicken breast tenders
- 24-oz pickle jar
- Salt and pepper, to taste
- ¼ cup grated Parmesan
- 2 large eggs
- 1 tsp paprika
- 2 tbsp avocado oil

Directions:
1. Take the pickles out from the jar.
2. Put the chicken in a plastic bag, then pour the pickle juice over it.
3. Put the chicken in the fridge and let it marinate for at least 1 hour.
4. Use a bowl to mix the grated Parmesan, protein powder, salt, pepper, and paprika, and whisk the eggs together on a separate plate.
5. Place a skillet on the stove over medium-high heat. Pour the avocado oil into the skillet. Then let it heat up while you bread the chicken.
6. First, cover the chicken tenders with the whisked eggs before coating them with the crumbly breading mixture.
7. Pan fry until the tenders are golden brown and fully cooked through.

Keto Roasted Pumpkin & Halloumi Salad

Time: 1 hour
Serving Size: 4 servings

Prep Time: 15 minutes

Cook Time: 45 minutes

Nutritional Facts/Info:

Calories 522

Carbs 21.5 g

Fat 42.3 g

Protein 19.8 g

Ingredients:
The Salad
- 1 tsp paprika
- 1 tbsp olive oil
- 1 ¼ cups diced pumpkin
- 1 tbsp butter
- salt, to taste
- 3 tbsps flaked almonds
- 4 oz halloumi, cubed
- 1/2 medium avocado, sliced
- 200 grams watercress

Dressing
- 1 tbsp lemon juice
- 1 tbsp olive oil
- 1 tsp tahini
- 1/8 tsp apple cider vinegar
- 1/8 tsp salt

Directions:
1. Preheat your oven to 400°F.
2. Combine the diced pumpkin along with the olive oil, paprika, and salt and layer it onto a baking tray then roast for 20 minutes or until it's brown and slightly soft.
3. Take out a nonstick pan and use it to melt the butter. Sauté the halloumi for 15 minutes, flipping it occasionally, until the cheese has started to look crisp and brown. Set aside.
4. Roast the almonds on a roasting tray for 6–10 minutes. Make sure that they are evenly spread out and give the tray a shake halfway through. Leave them for later once they are done.
5. Create the fresh dressing by mixing the tahini, olive oil, lemon juice, salt, and apple cider vinegar.
6. Arrange the roasted pumpkin, almonds, halloumi, and avocado over a bed of watercress tucked into a bowl before topping off with a decent helping of the dressing scattered over the top.

Keto Meaty Mediterranean Lunch Bowls

Time: 25 minutes
Serving Size: 5 servings

Prep Time: 10 minutes

Cook Time: 15 minutes

Nutritional Facts/Info:

Calories 502.2

Carbs 11.08 g

Fat 36.82 g

Protein 31.38 g

Ingredients:
Meatballs:
- 1 large egg
- 1 cup grated Parmesan cheese
- 1 lb ground chicken
- 1 tsp lemon zest
- 2 tsp Italian seasoning
- 1 clove garlic, minced
- 2 tbsps butter
- salt and pepper, to taste

Lunch Bowls:
- 1 large head of romaine lettuce

- 1 medium cucumber, peeled and sliced
- 1 large green bell pepper, sliced
- 1 ¼ cup cherry tomatoes, halved
- 5 tsp olive oil
- 1 small red onion, sliced

Tomato and Basil Dressing
- 1 tbsp unsweetened tomato paste
- ¼ cup mayonnaise
- ¼ cup sour cream
- 1 tbsp chopped basil
- 2 tbsps chopped sun-dried tomatoes
- salt and pepper, to taste
- ½ tbsp lemon juice

Directions:
1. Use a large mixing bowl to add the ground chicken, parmesan cheese, garlic, egg, Italian seasoning, lemon zest, salt, and pepper. Mix everything and then roll out 25 meatballs.
2. Heat some butter in a large skillet, over high heat. Once the butter has melted and the foaming has stopped, lower the heat to medium-high.
3. Pop the meatballs in, and brown them evenly and until they are cooked through. Remove them and let them drain on a paper towel.
4. Now it is ready to serve. Begin by dividing the lettuce leaves into bowls before adding in the fresh and juicy cucumbers, cherry tomatoes, bell pepper, red onion, and olive oil.
5. Place the remaining ingredients in a bowl and mix well to create the tomato and basil dressing.
6. 5 meatballs in each bowl should be enough with 3 tablespoons of dressing each.

Keto Crispy Ginger Mackerel Lunch Bowl

Time: 40 minutes
Serving Size: 2 servings

Prep Time: 20 minutes

Cook Time: 20 minutes

Nutritional Facts/Info:

Calories 649.55

Carbs 9.2 g

Fat 53.4 g

Protein 28.05 g

Ingredients:
Marinade:
- 3 tbsps olive oil
- 1 tbsp lemon juice
- 1 tbsp grated ginger
- salt and pepper, to taste
- 1 tbsp coconut aminos

Lunch bowl:
- 1 tbsp butter
- 1 oz almonds
- 2 (8-oz) boneless mackerel fillets
- 1 ½ cups broccoli

- 1/3 cup diced red bell pepper
- ½ small yellow onion
- 4 tbsps mashed avocado
- 2 small sun-dried tomatoes, chopped

Directions:
1. Preheat the oven to 400°F.
2. Cover a baking tray with foil to prepare for later.
3. Mix your grated ginger, olive oil, lemon juice, coconut aminos, and salt and pepper. Rub the mackerel fillets with only half of the marinade.
4. Place the fillets, skin side up, onto the baking tray.
5. Roast the mackerel for 12–15 minutes or until the skin crackles when you tap it, showing off a perfect crisp.
6. Place the almonds with adequate spacing between them on a separate baking sheet. Roast them for 5–6 minutes or until they slightly darken in color. Careful not to burn your fingers so allow them to cool before chopping them up.
7. Gently steam the broccoli until slightly soft to the touch but make sure it isn't mushy. Then roughly chop it up.
8. Preheat a pan over medium heat, and add the broccoli and sun-dried tomatoes, and cook briefly to heat them through.
9. Switch off the stove before pouring in the rest of the dressing and almonds.
10. Serve with the avocado, and enjoy!

Keto Bacon Cheeseburger Kebabs

Time: 30 minutes
Serving Size: 10 servings

Prep Time: 10 minutes

Cook Time: 20 minutes

Nutritional Facts/Info:

Calories 303.41

Carbs 3.29 g

Fat 23.4 g

Protein 18.45 g

Ingredients:
Kebabs
- 1 tsp black pepper
- 1 tbsp Worcestershire sauce
- 1 lb ground beef
- ½ tsp salt
- 1 tsp dried minced onion
- 1 tsp garlic powder
- 5 slices cheddar cheese, quartered
- 6 slices bacon
- 10 cherry tomatoes
- ½ head iceberg lettuce
- 20 slices dill pickles

Dipping Sauce:
- 2 tbsps minced onion
- 2 tbsps sugar-free ketchup
- ½ cup mayonnaise
- 1 tbsp mustard
- pickle juice, to taste
- 2 tbsps minced dill pickles

Directions:
1. Preheat the grill to 375°F.
2. Make sure that you can do both direct and indirect cooking.
3. Mix the ground beef, Worcestershire sauce, pepper, salt, garlic powder, and minced onion.
4. Then use a scoop to form even balls, then mold them into patties.
5. Use a cast-iron skillet. Place it over the indirect heat before cooking the bacon, leaving them soft and not letting them get crispy to enable you to skewer them. Leave the bacon on a plate and clean the pan.
6. Place the skillet back over the indirect heat and place the burger patties in the heated pan. Turn them halfway through the cooking time when the side starts to crisp and the aromas waft around the house.
7. Use large skewers to arrange the patties, bacon, tomatoes, lettuce, and pickle slices. There should be two patties per skewer.
8. Mix the remaining ingredients into a delicious dipping sauce or just pour some over your skewer.

Keto Tuna Cheese Melt

Time: 50 minutes
Serving Size: 2 servings

Prep Time: 10 minutes

Cook Time: 40 minutes

Nutritional Facts/Info:

Calories 787

Carbs 5 g

Fat 67 g

Protein 38 g

Ingredients:
bread
- 3 eggs
- 4½ oz cream cheese softened
- 1 pinch salt
- ½ tbsp ground psyllium husk powder
- ½ tsp baking powder

Tuna salad
- ¾ cup mayonnaise or sour cream
- 4 celery stalks, minced
- 2 oz dill pickles, chopped
- 8 oz tuna in water drained

- 1 tsp lemon juice
- 1 garlic clove, minced
- salt and pepper, to taste

Topping
- 10 oz shredded cheese
- ¼ tsp cayenne pepper or paprika powder

For serving
- 5 oz leafy greens
- olive oil

Directions:
Bread
1. Preheat the oven to 300°F.
2. Line a half-sheet pan, with parchment paper.
3. You'll want the egg whites away from the yolk, so divide them and place them into separate bowls.
4. A pinch of salt over the egg whites, before creating a stiff whip using the electric mixer. If you can turn the bowl around without the egg whites moving, you're done.
5. Entwine the egg yolks and cream cheese together using the electric mixer, and then stir in the psyllium husk and baking powder.
6. Fold the egg whites into the egg yolk mix gently, trying to keep the air in the egg whites.
7. Each serving requires 2 equal mounds of smooth batter, so divide these on the parchment-lined baking tray. Create ½" thick circles using a spatula.
8. The middle rack is best if you bake for about 25 minutes, until golden, then set aside to cool.

Tuna cheese melts
9. Preheat the oven to 350°F.

10. Mix the tuna salad ingredients.
11. Take the baking tray with the cooled bread, and spread a generous helping of tuna salad on top of each slice.
12. Sprinkle the cheese and cayenne, or paprika on top. Bake on the middle rack for about 15 minutes.
13. Serve the tuna melt on top of fresh leafy greens, drizzled with a dash of olive oil

Keto Thai Fish Curry

Time: 30 minutes
Serving Size: 1 serving

Prep Time: 10 minutes

Cook Time: 20 minutes

Nutritional Facts/Info:

Calories 1014

Carbs 10 g

Fat 90 g

Protein 42 g

Ingredients:
- 2 oz coconut oil for greasing the baking dish
- 1½ lbs salmon, boneless fillets or white fish, in pieces
- salt and pepper
- 2 oz butter or ghee
- 2 tbsp red curry paste or green curry paste
- 2 cups canned, unsweetened coconut cream
- ½ cup fresh cilantro, chopped
- 1 lb cauliflower or broccoli

Directions:
1. Preheat the oven to 400°F.
2. Grease a medium-sized baking dish.
3. Then place the fish pieces in the baking dish. Season with salt and pepper and top off each fish piece with a dollop of butter.
4. Mix up the coconut cream, curry paste, and chopped cilantro in a small bowl to pour over the fish.
5. Bake in the oven for 20 minutes until the fish starts to bubble golden brown.
6. While the fish is cooking, break up the cauliflower into florets and boil in lightly salted water until tender.
7. Serve, and enjoy!

Creamy Keto Fish Casserole

Time: 45 minutes
Serving Size: 4 servings

Prep Time: 15 minutes

Cook Time: 30 minutes

Nutritional Facts/Info:

Calories 804

Carbs 9 g

Fat 67 g

Protein 40 g

Ingredients:
- 2 tbsp olive oil
- 1 lb broccoli, small florets
- 1 oz butter, for greasing the casserole dish
- 2 tbsp small capers
- 4 oz scallions
- 1¼ cups heavy whipping cream
- 1½ lbs white fish, in serving-sized pieces
- 1 tsp salt
- 1 tbsp Dijon mustard
- 1 tbsp dried parsley
- ½ tsp ground black pepper
- 3 oz butter

For serving
- 5 oz leafy greens

Directions:
1. Preheat the oven to 400°F.
2. Cut the broccoli, including the stem.
3. Fry the broccoli in an oiled skillet on medium-high for 5 minutes, until golden and soft. Then season with salt and pepper.
4. Add the scallions, finely chopped, and the capers.
5. Fry for a further 1–2 minutes before arranging the vegetables in a greased baking dish.
6. Nestle the fish in amongst the vegetables.
7. Mix parsley, whipping cream, and mustard. Pour the mixture over the fish as well as the vegetables. Decorate it with slices of butter on top.
8. Bake for 20 minutes or until the fish is cooked through, and flakes easily.
9. Serve as is, or with a leafy salad.

Keto Meat Pie

Time: 1 hr 20 minutes
Serving Size: 1 serving

Prep Time: 15 minutes

Cook Time: 75 minutes

Nutritional Facts/Info:

Calories 546 | Carbs 6 g | Fat 42 g | Protein 33 g

Ingredients:
Filling
- ½ yellow onion, finely chopped
- 1 garlic clove, finely chopped
- 2 tbsp butter or olive oil
- 1¼ lbs ground beef or turkey
- 1 tbsp dried oregano or dried basil
- salt and pepper
- 3 tbsp tomato paste
- ½ cup water

Pie crust
- ¾ cup almond flour
- ¼ cup sesame seeds
- ¼ cup coconut flour
- 1 tbsp ground psyllium husk powder
- 1 tsp baking powder
- 1 pinch salt
- 3 tbsp olive oil
- 1 large egg
- ¼ cup water

Topping
- 1 cup cottage cheese
- 1 cup shredded cheese

Directions:
1. Preheat the oven to 350°F.
2. Fry up some onion and garlic in the oil of your choice over medium heat for a few minutes or until the onion is soft.
3. Add ground beef and keep frying. Then add oregano or basil and season with salt and pepper to taste.
4. Add tomato paste or if you would like some ajvar relish instead. But add water. Drop down the heat creating a simmer for at least 20 minutes.
5. While the meat simmers, use the time to make the dough for the crust.
6. Toss all the ingredients for the crust into a food processor for a few minutes until the dough becomes a ball.
7. Insert a rounded piece of parchment paper into a greased springform pan or deep-dish pie pan.
8. Cover the base of the pan with the dough and push it up the sides. A spatula works well for this or just some well-greased fingers. Once the crust is shaped nicely to fit the pan, prick the bottom of the crust with a fork.
9. Pre-bake the crust for 10–15 minutes. Then remove from the oven before pouring in the juicy meat.
10. Mix both the cottage cheese and shredded cheese to create a layer on top of the pie.
11. Bake on the lower rack for 30–40 minutes.

Keto Lasagna

Time: 1 hr 15 minutes
Serving Size: 1 serving

Prep Time: 15 minutes

Cook Time: 60 minutes

Nutritional Facts/Info:

Calories 756

Carbs 8 g

Fat 60 g

Protein 41 g

Ingredients:
Lasagna sheets
- 8 eggs, beaten
- 10 oz cream cheese
- 1 tsp salt
- 1/3 cup ground psyllium husk powder

Meat sauce
- 3 tbsp olive oil
- ½ yellow onion, finely chopped
- 1 garlic clove, finely chopped
- 1½ lbs ground beef
- 2 tbsp tomato paste

- ½ tbsp dried basil
- 1 tsp salt
- ¼ tsp ground black pepper
- ½ cup water

Cheese topping
- 1½ cups sour cream
- 1 cup shredded mozzarella cheese
- ½ cup shredded parmesan cheese
- ½ tsp salt
- ¼ tsp ground black pepper
- ½ cup fresh parsley, finely chopped

Directions:
Lasagna sheets
1. Preheat the oven to 300°F.
2. Line a baking sheet with parchment paper.
3. Use a medium-sized bowl to whisk together the ingredients, until a smooth batter forms. Then whisk in the psyllium husk, before placing it to the side for now.
4. If you want a thick paste, spread all the batter in the middle of the paper before placing more paper on top and flattening it with a rolling pin until the batter is at least 13" x 18". Unless you want a thinner pasta, you should then divide the batter into two equal batches, before flattening them out.
5. Bake each sheet (with parchment paper) for about 10-12 minutes then set aside to cool.
6. Now, peel off the paper before slicing the pasta batter into sheets that will fit snugly into a 9" x 12" baking dish.

Meat sauce
7. Use a large pan, over medium-high heat, to warm the olive oil.

8. Add the onion and garlic, stirring until soft.
9. Now add the beef, tomato paste, and spices, and combine thoroughly. Stop when you can't see any pinker on the beef.
10. Add water to the mixture, before bringing to a boil and then lower the heat, and let simmer for at least 15 minutes or until moist.
11. Preheat the oven to 400 degrees Fahrenheit and grease a 9" x 12" baking dish.

Cheese topping
12. Mix all of the cheese but only a little of the parmesan.
13. Layer the pasta sheets along with the meat sauce into the baking dish, starting with the pasta, followed by the meat sauce.
14. Lather the cheese mixture generously over the top of the pasta tower, and finish with the extra parmesan cheese.
15. Bake in the oven for about 30 minutes or until the lasagna has browned nicely.
16. Serve, and enjoy!

Keto Asian Cabbage Stir-Fry

Time: 20 minutes
Serving Size: 4 servings

Prep Time: 10 minutes

Cook Time: 10 minutes

Nutritional Facts/Info:

Calories 943

Carbs 9 g

Fat 86 g

Protein 31 g

Ingredients:
- 1 tsp salt
- 4 oz butter, divided
- 1 lb green cabbage
- ¼ tsp ground black pepper
- 1 tsp onion powder
- 2 garlic cloves, minced
- 1 tbsp white wine vinegar
- 2 oz fresh ginger, finely chopped or grated
- 1 tsp chili flakes
- 3 scallions, chopped in 1/2" (2.5 cm) slices
- 1¼ lbs ground beef
- 1 tbsp sesame oil

Wasabi mayonnaise
- ½ tbsp wasabi paste
- 1 cup mayonnaise

Directions:
1. Finely slice the cabbage using a sharp knife or a food processor.
2. Using a wok pan, fry the cabbage over medium or high heat until softened. Do not let it brown.
3. Then add spices and vinegar. Stir fry the vegetable for a touch longer before pouring it into a heat-resistant bowl.
4. Melt the rest of the butter in the same used wok and add garlic, chili flakes, and ginger. Sauté everything for a few minutes.
5. Mix in some ground meat cooking all the way through, giving the meat a sizzling brown look.
6. Now add scallions and cabbage to the meat, stirring till everything is hot.
7. Spice up the meal with some salt and pepper and sesame oil before serving. As well as the wasabi mayonnaise created by adding a small amount of wasabi to the mayo and adding more until the flavor is just right.
8. Serve, and enjoy!

Italian Keto Meatballs with Mozzarella Cheese

Time: 30 minutes
Serving Size: 1 serving

Prep Time: 10 minutes

Cook Time: 20 minutes

Nutritional Facts/Info:

Calories 630

Carbs 5 g

Fat 49 g

Protein 40 g

Ingredients:
- 1 lb ground beef
- ¾ cup shredded Parmesan cheese
- 1 egg
- 1 tsp salt
- ½ tbsp dried basil
- ½ tsp onion powder
- 1 tsp garlic powder
- ½ tsp ground black pepper
- 3 tbsp olive oil
- 1¾ cups canned whole tomatoes
- 2 tbsp fresh parsley, finely chopped
- 7 oz fresh spinach

- 2 oz butter
- 5 oz fresh mozzarella cheese
- salt and pepper

Directions:
1. Place ground beef, egg, parmesan cheese, salt, and spices in a bowl and blend.
2. Wet your hands and form the mixture into meatballs, about 1 oz each. You can either wet your hands with water or moisten them with olive oil.
3. Use a large skillet to heat the olive oil and sauté the meatballs until they're completely browned all over.
4. Drop down the heat before pouring in the canned tomatoes, letting them simmer bubbly softly for 15 minutes, stir when the bubbles get erratic and turn down the heat if it begins bubbling.
5. Season with salt and pepper to taste. Add parsley and stir.
6. Prepare the butter in a different pan and sizzle up the spinach for 1–2 minutes, stirring continuously.
7. Season with salt and pepper to taste. Combine the spinach with the meatballs and meld the meat and veggie flavors together.
8. Serve with mozzarella cheese on top and enjoy!

Easy Low-Carb Cauliflower Mac 'n Cheese

Time: 40 mins
Serving Size: 4 servings

Prep Time: 15 mins

Cook Time: 25 mins

Nutritional Facts/Info:

Calories 389

Carbs 9.5 g

Fat 35 g

Protein 12 g

Ingredients:
- 1 head cauliflower, cut into florets
- 1 tsp salt
- 1 tsp mixed herbs
- ½ tsp ground black pepper
- 3 tbsp olive oil
- 1 cup shredded cheddar cheese
- ½ cup heavy whipping cream
- 1 tbsp ghee (clarified butter)
- 1 pinch ground nutmeg
- 3 tbsps grated parmesan cheese

Directions:
1. Preheat the oven to 450°F.
2. Line a baking sheet with aluminum foil.
3. Arrange the cauliflower on the prepared baking sheet, then sprinkle it with salt, mixed herbs, and pepper, and drizzle some olive oil on it; toss until well coated.
4. Place the baking sheet with cauliflower in the preheated oven and roast until crisp (this should take about 10 to 15 minutes).
5. Transfer the baked cauliflower into an 8-inch baking dish and set aside.
6. Combine cheddar cheese, heavy cream, ghee, and nutmeg in a saucepan over medium heat.
7. Allow the mixture to simmer until bubbly, about 5 minutes. Then pour over the cauliflower and mix well. Sprinkle parmesan cheese on top.
8. Bake in the preheated oven until golden for about 10 minutes.
9. Serve, and enjoy!

Cobb Salad

Time: 50 mins
Serving Size: 6 servings

Prep Time: 20 mins

Cook Time: 30 mins

Nutritional Facts/Info:

Calories 525

Carbs 10.2 g

Fat 39.9 g

Protein 31.7 g

Ingredients:
- 6 slices bacon
- 3 eggs
- 1 head iceberg lettuce, shredded
- 3 cups chopped, cooked chicken meat
- 2 tomatoes, seeded and chopped
- ¾ cup blue cheese, crumbled
- 1 avocado, peeled, pitted, and diced
- 3 green onions, chopped
- 1 (8 ounces) bottle ranch-style salad dressing

Directions:
1. Place the eggs in a saucepan and cover completely with cold water.
2. Bring water to a boil.
3. Cover and remove from heat, then let eggs stand in hot water for 10 to 12 minutes.
4. Remove the boiled eggs from hot water, wait for them to cool, peel and chop.
5. Use a deep skillet to cook the bacon over medium-high heat. Wait for the bacon to become evenly brown, then drain it from the oil, crumble it and set it aside.
6. Divide the shredded lettuce among individual plates.
7. Evenly divide and arrange chicken, eggs, tomatoes, blue cheese, bacon, avocado, and green onions in a row on top of the lettuce.
8. Drizzle your favorite dressing and enjoy.

Keto Instant Pot Soup (Low Carb)

Time: 58 mins
Serving Size: 6 servings

Prep Time: 20 mins

Cook Time: 33 mins

Nutritional Facts/Info:

Calories 347

Carbs 13.4 g

Fat 25.6 g

Protein 17.7 g

Ingredients:
- 1 tablespoon olive oil
- 1 large yellow onion, diced
- 2 cloves garlic, minced
- 1 head cauliflower, coarsely chopped
- 1 green bell pepper, chopped (optional)
- 1 tbsp onion powder
- salt and ground black pepper to taste
- 1 (32 fluid oz) container chicken stock
- 2 cups shredded cheddar cheese
- 1 cup half-and-half
- 6 slices cooked turkey bacon, diced
- 1 tbsp Dijon mustard

- 4 dashes of hot pepper sauce

Directions:
1. Turn on a multi-cooker and select the sauté function.
2. Add some olive oil, onion, and garlic; cook until browned for about 3 minutes.
3. Add the cauliflower, green bell pepper, onion powder, and season with salt and pepper.
4. Pour in the chicken stock; close and lock the lid.
5. Now select the Soup function and set the timer for 15 minutes. Allow the pressure to build for around 10 or possibly 15 minutes.
6. Take extra care when releasing the pressure using the quick-release method and take note to follow the manufacturer's instructions, which is about 5 minutes.
7. Unlock and remove the lid.
8. Add cheddar cheese, half-and-half, tasty turkey bacon, spicy Dijon mustard, and hot sauce. Put it back in the sauté function; cook until bubbly, about 5 minutes.
9. Serve, and enjoy!

Easy Keto Beef Tacos

Time: 50 mins
Serving Size: 4 servings

Prep Time: 20 mins

Cook Time: 18 mins

Nutritional Facts/Info:

Calories 676

Carbs 9.7 g

Fat 52.6 g

Protein 40.7 g

Ingredients:
- 2 cups shredded cheddar cheese
- 1 lb ground beef
- ½ package taco seasoning mix
- ½ tsp salt
- ¼ tsp ground black pepper
- 1 avocado, diced
- 1 cup shredded lettuce
- ½ cup shredded cheddar cheese
- ½ cup tomatoes, diced

Directions:
1. Preheat the oven to 350°F.
2. Line 2 baking sheets using parchment paper or a more sustainable option is silicone mats.
3. Spread cheddar cheese into four 6-inch circles.
4. Bake in the preheated oven until the cheese melts and is slightly brown, (this should take about 6 to 8 minutes).
5. Cool for 2 to 3 minutes before lifting with a spatula.
6. Place the tacos over a wooden spoon handle wrapped in aluminum foil balanced over 2 cups/cans. Let taco shells cool completely, about 10 minutes.
7. Cook beef in a skillet over medium-high heat until browned, stirring often to separate meat, about 7 minutes.
8. Season with taco seasoning, salt, and pepper; cook for 1 minute more.
9. Divide beef mixture among cheese taco shells.
10. Top with avocado, lettuce, cheddar cheese, and tomatoes.

Caveman Chili

Time: 6 hours 35 minutes
Serving Size: 8 servings

Prep Time: 20 mins

Cook Time: 6 hrs 15 mins

Nutritional Facts/Info:

Calories 357

Carbs 22 g

Fat 12.2 g

Protein 27.4 g

Ingredients:
- 1 (14.5 oz) can diced tomatoes, drained
- 8 thick slices bacon, chopped
- 2 pounds ground pork
- 3 small green bell peppers, chopped
- 1 onion, chopped
- 1 (1.25 oz) package chili seasoning (such as McCormick®)
- 1 (6 oz) can tomato paste
- 1 pinch onion powder, or more to taste
- 1 pinch garlic powder, or more to taste
- salt and ground black pepper to taste
- 1 pinch ground cayenne pepper, or more to taste

Directions:
1. Place the pork in a skillet on medium heat before seasoning with salt and pepper.
2. Cook and stir until browned and crumbly, this should roughly take 5 to 7 minutes.
3. Drain the grease and discard it. Then transfer the pork to a slow cooker.
4. Use a hot oiled skillet to brown the bacon evenly for about 10 minutes.
5. Drain and discard grease then transfer bacon to the slow cooker.
6. Drain the tomatoes before adding the onion, tomato paste, and green bell pepper.
7. Sprinkle in all the spices in the combinations you prefer.
8. Cook on Low until flavors have combined, about 6 hours.
9. Serve, and enjoy!

Seafood Stuffed Avocados

Time: 15 mins
Serving Size: 2 servings

Prep Time: 15 mins

Nutritional Facts/Info:

Calories 283

Carbs 10 g

Fat 21.1 g

Protein 16.5 g

Ingredients:
- 1 tbsp mayonnaise
- ½ cup cooked small shrimp
- ½ cup flaked cooked crabmeat
- 2 tbsp peeled and diced cucumber
- 1 pinch salt
- 1 tsp chopped fresh parsley
- 1 pinch paprika
- 1 pinch ground black pepper
- 1 avocado

Directions:
1. Use a bowl to mix the crab, shrimp, cucumber, mayonnaise, and parsley.
2. Season with salt, and pepper.
3. Cover, and chill till it is time to serve.

4. Slice the avocados into long strips, and throw away the pit.
5. Scoop out the flesh of the avocado leaving an approximate 1/2-inch layer cradled in the peel.
6. Pack the hollowed centers of the avocado halves with the seafood mixture.
7. Sprinkle the tops with paprika.
8. Serve, and enjoy!

Chapter 5: Keto Dinner Recipes

Delicious Keto Recipes

Easy Chicken Cordon Bleu Casserole

This hearty zucchini and chicken meal is baked in a creamy three-cheese sauce that will keep taste buds charmed. It is tasty enough to prepare for family members who are not on the diet with you.

Time: 1 hour 15 minutes
Serving Size: 4 servings

Prep Time: 20 minutes

Cook Time: 55 minutes

Nutritional Facts/Info:

Calories 373 | Carbs 8 g | Fat 26 g | Protein 27 g

Ingredients:
- 2 large cloves garlic crushed
- 1/2 small onion diced
- 1 tbsp unsalted butter
- 4 oz cream cheese at room temperature
- 1 cup chicken bone broth
- 2 tbsps chopped fresh parsley

- 2 oz Emmental cheese shredded (or Swiss cheese)
- 1/8 tsp black pepper
- 1/2 tsp Worcestershire sauce
- 2 cups cooked shredded chicken
- 1 lb zucchini sliced
- 2 tbsps grated Parmesan
- 2 tbsps cured pork belly crisped

Directions:
1. Preheat the oven to 375°F before preparing a 1.5-quart casserole dish for later.
2. In a skillet on the stovetop, melt the butter over medium heat and then add the onions. Stir the onions for around 3 minutes, allowing them to soften but not brown. Mix in the garlic for 1 minute, treating it the same as the onion.
3. Incorporate the broth in the pan and let it simmer. Fold in the cream cheese mixture until a smooth mix is created; let it simmer for a couple of minutes. As it thickens, whisk frequently.
4. Toss the Emmental cheese into the mix a handful at a time until it melts into the sauce. Sprinkle in the parsley, then pour in the Worcestershire, and black pepper. Stir before taking it off the heat.
5. Gently lay the chicken and then the zucchini into the casserole dish and cover with the creamy sauce. Take pinches of the crisped pork belly and sprinkle over the chicken followed by a sprinkle of Parmesan.
6. Encase the dish with tin foil to lock in the steamy flavors and bake for 45 minutes or until the chicken is cooked thoroughly.
7. Strip off the foil and allow the dish to boil for a few minutes to brown the top.
8. Serve.

Low-Carb Keto Indian Butter Chicken

Time: 1 hour
Serving Size: 4 servings

Prep Time: 25 minutes

Cook Time: 35 minutes

Nutritional Facts/Info:

Calories 469 | Carbs 9.8 g | Fat 31 g | Protein 37.7 g

Ingredients:
- 1/2 tsp turmeric
- 1 tsp cumin
- 1 tbsp garam masala spice mix
- 1/2 tsp coriander
- 1/4 tsp cinnamon
- 1/4 tsp black pepper
- 1/4 tsp fenugreek

For the Chicken
- 1/2 tsp sea salt
- 2 tsp spice mix from recipe above
- 1 lb chicken breast skinless
- 2 tbsps fresh lemon juice
- 2 large cloves garlic crushed
- 3 tbsps sour cream

Sauce:
- 1-inch piece fresh ginger grated
- 1 medium yellow onion diced
- 4 tbsps ghee

- 3 cloves garlic crushed
- 1/2 tsp sea salt
- remaining spice mix from the recipe above
- 1 1/2 cups low-sodium chicken bone broth or water
- 1/4 tsp crushed red pepper flakes more or less to taste
- 1/2 cup grass-fed heavy whipping cream
- 4 tsp tomato paste

For serving (optional):
- A small handful of fresh cilantro leaves
- Sliced red onion

Directions:
1. Combine all the spices to create your tangy spice mix.
2. The chicken can be prepared ahead of time, perhaps up to two days before. Toss all the chicken ingredients in a bowl allowing the flavors to seep into the chicken.
3. Leave the chicken in the fridge for at least 2 hours before cooking in a preheated oven set to 400° F. This should take up to 15 minutes. It's ready when it is no longer pink in the middle.
4. Begin the sauce by heating the ghee in a deep skillet using medium heat. Toss in the onion, stirring frequently until the onion releases its sugar and begins to create a caramelized coating, roughly 20 minutes. Combine the ginger, garlic, and spice mix for one minute before adding in the rest of the ingredients and bringing to a boil. Reduce to simmer for 10 minutes, before letting it cool down enough to be blended.
5. Pour it back into the pan before adding the chicken and whipping cream.
6. Sprinkle fresh cilantro and sliced red onion, on top to garnish, if desired.

Cheese Fathead Pizza Crust

Time: 15 minutes
Serving Size: 8 slices

Prep Time: 5 minutes

Cook Time: 10 minutes

Nutritional Facts/Info:

Calories 334

Carbs 6 g

Fat 27 g

Protein 17 g

Ingredients:
Pizza Dough:
- 1 tsp psyllium husk powder
- 2 tbsps warm water
- 1 tsp instant yeast
- 1 cup almond flour
- 1 1/2 cups shredded low-moisture part-skim mozzarella
- 1 tsp baking powder
- 1 large egg beaten
- 1 oz cream cheese
- Avocado oil olive oil, or ghee, for oiling your hands

Garlic Cream Sauce:
- 1 tbsp heavy whipping cream
- 2 large cloves garlic crushed or minced
- 2 tbsps unsalted butter
- 3 oz cream cheese
- 1/8 tsp salt
- 1 tsp dried parsley flakes
- 1/8 tsp black pepper

Other:
- 6 oz shredded mozzarella cheese
- 2 tsp minced fresh parsley for garnish
- 3 oz shredded white cheddar cheese

Directions:
1. A clay baking stone works perfectly to create the soft and crispy base but preheating an oven to 425°F without the stone works well, too.
2. Create a pool of warm water in a bowl before adding in the yeast. Stir. Leaving it for around 5 to 10 minutes lets the foam begin to form.
3. The almond flour, baking powder, and psyllium husk powder need to be combined in a separate bowl.
4. Microwave the two kinds of cheese in a heat-resistant bowl by first giving it a 60-second boost, followed by 20-second bursts until the two kinds of cheese combine to form a melted masterpiece.
5. Add the yeast and beaten eggs to the bowl, combining well before the almond flour is added. This makes the dough.
6. Oil your hands before kneading the dough and creating a ball.
7. Roll out the ball into your desired pizza size. Using two pieces of parchment paper helps to keep the dough

from sticking to your hands. Create small holes all around the circle using a fork.
8. Place the prepared dough into the oven or onto the stove and watch it turn golden in spots, this should only take 6 minutes and should not cook fully. If the baking stone was not available, the cookie sheet will work well but you will need to cook for 8 minutes.
9. The base will be needed to assemble the pizza while the oven should stay heated at 425°F.
10. The garlic sauce can be created when the base is being heated by melted butter in a skillet, adding garlic for a minute, and then the rest of the sauce ingredients until thick and smooth.
11. Start assembling the pizza by spreading the sauce evenly and generously over the base before adding the desired amount of cheese, both mozzarella, and cheddar.
12. The pizza is ready to bake in the oven for another 7 minutes or until the bubbling cheese is too perfect to resist any longer.
13. Sprinkle the parsley on top and serve

Beef Chili Recipe (Beanless Chili)

Time: 55 minutes
Serving Size: 8 people

Prep Time: 15 minutes

Cook Time: 40 minutes

Nutritional Facts/Info:

Calories 405

Carbs 8 g

Fat 30 g

Protein 25 g

Ingredients:
- 2 tbsps avocado oil
- 1 lb 85% lean ground beef
- 1 lb Italian sausage (hot or mild; bulk or removed from casing)
- 6 large cloves garlic crushed
- 6 large stalks celery chopped
- 1 medium yellow onion chopped
- 5 cups beef bone broth
- 6 oz tomato paste
- 1 tbsp chili powder
- 1/2 tbsp dried oregano
- 1 tsp cumin

- 1/2 tsp turmeric
- 1/4 tsp black pepper
- Fresh cilantro for serving (optional)

Directions:
1. Turn the pressure cooker on, press "Sauté", and wait 2 minutes for the pot to heat up. Add the oil, beef, and sausage, and cook until browned, about 3 to 5 minutes, stirring occasionally to break up the meat. Add the garlic until soft, usually about a minute, stirring constantly. Press "Cancel" to stop sautéing.
2. Stir in the celery, onion, broth, tomato paste, chili powder, oregano, cumin, turmeric, and black pepper. Turn the pot on Manual, High Pressure for 5 minutes, and then do a quick release.
3. Serve garnished with fresh cilantro if desired.

Easy Keto Bacon Cheeseburger Skillet.

Time: 1 hour
Serving Size: 6 servings

Prep Time: 15 minutes

Cook Time: 45 minutes

Nutritional Facts/Info:

Calories 606

Carbs 5 g

Fat 44 g

Protein 45 g

Ingredients:
- 1 ½ lb. ground beef
- ½ medium onion chopped
- ½ cup crumbled bacon pieces
- 2 tbsp sugar-free ketchup
- 1 tbsp Dijon mustard
- 2 tsp chopped fresh dill
- 1 tbsp Worcestershire sauce
- 3 oz cream cheese
- 2 tsp minced garlic
- 4 large eggs
- salt and pepper to taste
- 1 ½ cup cheddar cheese shredded

- ⅓ cup heavy whipping cream

Directions:
1. Preheat the oven to 350°F.
2. Take a large skillet and heat it over medium-high heat, cook the ground beef and onions until the ground beef is fully browned and the onions get slightly soft.
3. Reduce the heat to medium.
4. Throw in the ketchup, Worcestershire sauce, mustard, dill, minced garlic, cream cheese and sprinkle salt and pepper to taste. Stir everything together to combine and the melted cheese incorporates into all the ingredients.
5. Take the meat mixture and place it in a layer evenly measured out in a 9" x 13" baking dish, then scatter the crumbled bacon pieces on top.
6. Now, take a small bowl and whisk together the eggs and heavy whipping cream. Drizzle the mixture slowly and evenly over the meat in the baking dish.
7. Shredded cheddar cheese is a must to top it off.
8. Bake for 30–35 minutes until everything is cooked through and browned and bubbling.
9. If you want a touch of freshness, add some freshly chopped parsley as a garnish.
10. Serve, and enjoy!

Keto Skillet Chicken in Lemon Cream Sauce

Time: 40 minutes
Serving Size: 5 servings

Prep Time: 15 minutes

Cook Time: 25 minutes

Nutritional Facts/Info:

Calories 348

Carbs 9 g

Fat 17 g

Protein 39 g

Ingredients:
- 4 thin-cut boneless skinless chicken breast cutlets
- 1 cup bone broth
- 2 tbsp. olive oil
- 3 tsp. minced garlic
- a squeeze of fresh lemon juice to taste
- 1 tsp. Italian seasoning
- 1 diced shallot
- freshly chopped parsley for garnish
- ⅓ cup heavy whipping cream

Directions:
1. In a large skillet, heat olive oil over medium-high heat.
2. Now, season the chicken with salt and pepper flipping to do the same to the other side, and place it into the large heated skillet. Cook thoroughly by flipping it to evenly brown both sides.
3. Once the chicken is cooked, remove it from the skillet and set it aside.
4. Add the shallot to the pan and sauté for a few minutes.
5. Squeeze lemon juice in the skillet and add the minced garlic. Continue the sauté for 30 more seconds.
6. To create a slightly thick sauce, simply add the cream, Italian seasoning, and bone broth, stirring until the flavors have mixed.
7. Add the chicken to the skillet again, and pour the sauce mixture over the top of it.
8. Place some chopped parsley on top to garnish.
9. Serve, and enjoy!

Keto Buffalo Chicken Quesadilla

Time: 25 minutes
Serving Size: 3 servings

Prep Time: 10 minutes

Cook Time: 15 minutes

Nutritional Facts/Info:

Calories 404

Carbs 6 g

Fat 27 g

Protein 33 g

Ingredients:
- 1 cup shredded cheddar cheese
- 1 cup shredded mozzarella cheese
- 1/4 cup Frank's Red-Hot Sauce
- 2 tbsp melted butter
- 1 cup shredded cooked chicken

Directions:
1. Preheat the oven to 400°F.
2. Then mix all the mozzarella and cheddar cheeses, and form into a large circle on a parchment-lined baking sheet.

3. Bake the cheese for 10 minutes until it starts to brown on the edges, and it has taken on a lacelike appearance.
4. Now pour some olive oil into a skillet and heat over medium heat.
5. Add some red onions to the skillet, and cook until they start to soften.
6. Now place the shredded chicken in the skillet, and add some hot sauce. Then flip to coat.
7. Season with salt and pepper to taste.
8. Then, remove the cheese from the oven, and let sit aside to cool for a minute or two.
9. Distribute the chicken mixture in an even layer on one half of the cheese circle.
10. Then fold the other half of the cheese circle over the top of the filling, and bake for an additional 3-5 minutes.
11. Let sit to cool for several minutes before serving.
12. Serve, and enjoy!

Keto Bacon Cheeseburger Casserole

Time: 40 minutes
Serving Size: 1 serving

Prep Time: 15 minutes

Cook Time: 25 minutes

Nutritional Facts/Info:

Calories 484

Carbs 4 g

Fat 36 g

Protein 34 g

Ingredients:
- 1 tbsp olive oil
- 1 ½ lbs ground beef
- ½ cup onion, chopped
- 1 tsp oregano
- 2 tsp minced garlic
- 2 tsp Worcestershire sauce
- 2 tbsp sugar-free ketchup
- 3 oz cream cheese
- salt and pepper to taste
- 2 eggs
- ⅓ cup heavy whipping cream
- 2 cup shredded cheddar cheese, divided

- ½ cup pickle chips
- ½ cup bacon pieces

Directions:
1. Preheat the oven to 400°F.
2. Use an ovenproof skillet to heat the olive oil over a medium-heat stove.
3. Now, add the ground beef and onion to the skillet, and cook until the onion is slightly soft and the ground beef is browned.
4. Drain any excess grease, if needed.
5. Now, add the minced garlic, oregano, Worcestershire sauce, sugar-free ketchup, cream cheese, and salt and pepper to taste. Stir well.
6. Layer the meat mixture in the bottom of a casserole dish.
7. Use a small bowl to combine the eggs, heavy whipping cream, and a cup of cheese.
8. Pour the egg mixture over the top of the meat in the casserole dish.
9. Top the meat with a layer of pickle chips and then the crumbled bacon. Then sprinkle some extra cheese on top.
10. Bake for 20–25 minutes.
11. Serve with freshly chopped parsley and enjoy!

Keto Italian Cheese Stuffed Meatloaf

Time: 45 minutes
Serving Size: 1 serving

Prep Time: 15 minutes

Cook Time: 30 minutes

Nutritional Facts/Info:

Calories 511

Carbs 5 g

Fat 32 g

Protein 48 g

Ingredients:
- 2 lb ground beef
- 1 egg beaten
- ½ cup pork rind crumbs
- 1 small onion, chopped
- 1 tsp garlic powder
- 1 tsp Italian seasoning
- salt and pepper to taste
- 3 tbsp tomato paste
- 1 ¼ cups shredded mozzarella cheese divided
- ¼ cups low carb marinara sauce

Directions:
1. Preheat the oven to 350°F.
2. Use a large mixing bowl, combine the 2 pounds of ground beef with one small chopped onion. Use your hands to mix well.
3. Then, add in a beaten egg and ⅓ of a cup of pork rinds that have been made into very fine crumbs.
4. Now, sprinkle in 1 teaspoon of garlic powder and 1 teaspoon of Italian seasoning, add salt and pepper to taste.
5. Add 3 tablespoons of tomato paste into the bowl, and mix the ingredients well. Don't be shy about using your hands as this will bring about the best results.
6. Form the meat mixture into two smaller oval-shaped loaves. The small size will help them cook faster and thoroughly.
7. Make a divot down the center of each oval loaf of meat. Then, place a ½ cup of mozzarella cheese into the center of each meatloaf, and close the extra meat up over it, in this way, the cheese should be closed in the center of the loaves.
8. Top the meatloaves with a ¼ of a cup of low-carb marinara sauce.
9. Bake the meatloaves in a casserole dish for 30 minutes.
10. Remove the meatloaves, and top with ¼ cup of shredded mozzarella cheese. Return them to the oven and cook for an additional 5-10 minutes until the cheese is bubbly and the meat is cooked through.
11. Slice as desired. Serve and enjoy!

Keto Jalapeno Popper Stuffed Chicken

Time: 45 minutes
Serving Size: 1 serving

Prep Time: 10 minutes

Cook Time: 35 minutes

Nutritional Facts/Info:

Calories 503

Carbs 0 g

Fat 29 g

Protein 54 g

Ingredients:
- 2 oz cheddar jack shredded cheese
- 4 large jalapeno peppers
- 4 boneless skinless chicken breasts
- 4 oz cream cheese
- 4 tbsp almond flour
- 1 egg, beaten
- 1.5 oz crushed pork rind crumbs

Directions:
1. Preheat the oven to 400°F.
2. Cut a lengthwise little pocket in each chicken breast using a sharp knife. Be careful not to slice all the way

through. Make an incision that will allow you some room to put stuffing.

3. Create a creamy paste by mixing the cream cheese and the cheddar jack cheese with a fork in a medium-sized mixing bowl.
4. Cut the stems off the jalapeno peppers, then slice them in half lengthwise and use a spoon to remove and discard the seeds.
5. Encase the cheese filling in the spicy pepper by stuffing one half of the pepper full of cheese filling until it creates a mound and then closes it up with the other half of the pepper, creating a whole pepper once more.
6. Each chicken breast should encase a pepper, so place one in each pocket on the chicken breasts and fold the chicken around it. It may be hard to get the breast to close, so you can use a toothpick to hold the breast together.
7. Place the beaten egg in a shallow bowl, the almond flour on one plate, and the crushed pork rind crumbs on another.
8. Drench the chicken in the mix by creating a chain by dipping them in the almond flour, then the egg, and finally the crushed pork rind.
9. Season the chicken breasts with a pinch of salt and pepper.
10. The chicken cooks best on a baking rack or sheet for around 25 or 35 minutes. Make sure that there are no pink bits inside and the outside should have a crisp brown look.
11. Remove the breasts from the tray, place them on a serving dish and enjoy!

Keto Chicken Parmesan

Time: 28 minutes
Serving Size: 2 servings

Prep Time: 20 minutes

Cook Time: 8 minutes

Nutritional Facts/Info:

Calories 442

Carbs 5.8 g

Fat 25.3 g

Protein 46.5 g

Ingredients:
- 4 thin-cut chicken breasts
- 2 tbsp olive oil
- 1 cup crushed pork rind crumbs
- ¾ cup Parmesan cheese divided
- ½ tsp garlic powder
- 1 tsp basil
- Salt and pepper to taste
- ¼ c heavy whipping cream
- 1 egg, beaten
- 1 ½ cups low carb marinara sauce
- 1 ½ cups mozzarella cheese shredded

Directions:
1. Coat the thin-cut chicken breasts with 1 tsp of basil, as well as salt and pepper to taste. Make sure that you coat both sides.
2. Take a shallow bowl and place 1 beaten egg, and whisk in ¼ cup of heavy whipping cream.
3. Put 1 cup of crushed pork rind crumbs on a plate.
4. Mix ½ cup of grated Parmesan cheese and 1 tsp of garlic powder into the crushed pork rinds.
5. Use a large skillet to heat 2 tbsp of olive oil on medium-high heat.
6. Dip each chicken breast to drench it in the egg mixture, and then roll them in the crushed pork rind mixture to coat both sides.
7. Place the coated chicken breasts into the heated oil in the skillet. Cook evenly on both sides.
8. Turn the heat off to the burner, and heat the griller function on your oven.
9. Pour 1 ½ cups of low-carb marinara sauce over top of the cooked chicken in the skillet.
10. Top each piece of chicken with mozzarella cheese.
11. Put the skillet into the oven under the griller until the cheese is browned and bubbly.
12. Sprinkle ¼ cup of Parmesan cheese on top of the chicken.
13. Server, and enjoy!

Keto Ham and Cheese Crustless Quiche

Time: 1 hour
Serving Size: 4 servings

Prep Time: 15 minutes

Cook Time: 45 minutes

Nutritional Facts/Info:

Calories 979

Carbs 15.9 g

Fat 71.7 g

Protein 66.8 g

Ingredients:
- 5 eggs
- 1 cup heavy whipping cream
- 5 oz cubed ham
- ½ cup diced onion
- 1 scallion, chopped
- 2 cloves minced garlic
- salt and pepper to taste
- ½ cup Mozzarella cheese shredded
- 1 cup cheddar cheese shredded

Directions:
1. Firstly, preheat the oven to 350°F.
2. Place an oven-safe skillet on top of a medium heat stove to heat it.
3. Add the cubed ham into the heated skillet and sauté for about 2-3 minutes.
4. Now add in the garlic and scallions, and cook for 30 seconds more before removing the skillet from the heat.
5. Mix the eggs and heavy whipping cream in a bowl.
6. Then pour the egg and cream mixture over the meat in the skillet.
7. Sprinkle some salt and pepper to taste.
8. Sprinkle on the mozzarella and cheddar cheeses.
9. Finally, place the skillet into the oven, and bake for 35-40 minutes until the eggs are cooked through.

Keto Garlic Dusted Dinner Rolls

Time: 45 minutes
Serving Size: 8 servings

Prep Time: 30 minutes

Cook Time: 15 minutes

Nutritional Facts/Info:

Calories 282

Carbs 9 g

Fat 25.5 g

Protein 7.9 g

Ingredients:
- 1 ½ cup mozzarella cheese
- 1 ½ cup almond flour
- 2 oz cream cheese
- ½ tsp baking soda
- ½ tsp baking powder
- pinch of salt
- ¼ tsp Xanthan gum
- melted butter for brushing on the finished rolls
- 1 large egg
- garlic powder for dusting

Directions:
1. Preheat the oven to 350°F.
2. Place the cream cheese and mozzarella cheese in a heat-resistant bowl. Heat until the cheese is melted, roughly 1 ½ minute. When the cheese has melted, transfer to a mixing bowl.
3. Beat in the almond flour, baking powder, baking soda, xanthan gum, and a pinch of salt.
4. Then, add 1 egg, and mix well.
5. Encase the dough in plastic wrap, and refrigerate for 30 minutes.
6. Create 8 rounded balls of equal size by dividing the dough and rolling. Bake them on parchment paper for 12 minutes.
7. Remove the rolls from the oven, then grease the tops of the rolls with melted butter, and pour on a dusting of garlic powder. Pop bake in the oven for another 2 minutes.
8. Remove.
9. These are the tastiest when eaten warm, but you can also let them cool and store them in the fridge for another day.

Keto One Skillet Chicken in Lemon Cream Sauce

Time: 40 minutes
Serving Size: 2 servings

Prep Time: 10 minutes

Cook Time: 30 minutes

Nutritional Facts/Info:

Calories 495

Carbs 5.2 g

Fat 25.2 g

Protein 62.9 g

Ingredients:
- 4 thin-cut boneless skinless chicken breast cutlets
- 1 cup bone broth
- a squeeze of fresh lemon juice to taste
- 2 tbsp olive oil
- 1 diced shallot
- 3 tsp minced garlic
- ⅓ cup heavy whipping cream
- freshly chopped parsley for garnish
- 1 tsp Italian seasoning

Directions:
1. Using a large skillet placed on medium heat, warm up the olive oil.
2. Cover both sides of the chicken with salt and pepper, and place it into the large skillet.
3. Cook the chicken evenly on both sides until the heat has cooked it all the way through.
4. Take the chicken out of the skillet and let it rest.
5. Add some shallot to the pan and sauté for a few minutes.
6. Squeeze lemon juice to taste in the skillet and add the minced garlic.
7. Sauté for about 30 seconds longer.
8. Now, the bone broth, Italian seasoning, and heavy whipping cream should be poured into the skillet and cooked until the mixture thickens up nicely.
9. Add the chicken back to the skillet again, and drizzle the sauce mixture over the chicken.
10. Top with chopped parsley for garnish.
11. Serve, and enjoy!

Keto Mexican Zucchini and Beef

Time: 55 minutes
Serving Size: 6 servings

Prep Time: 10 minutes

Cook Time: 45 minutes

Nutritional Facts/Info:

Calories 819

Carbs 11 g

Fat 64 g

Protein 50 g

Ingredients:
- 1 ½ lbs ground beef
- 1 can Rotel
- 3 tsp minced garlic
- 2 small zucchinis, chopped
- 1 tsp cumin
- 1 tbsp chili powder
- ½ tsp oregano
- salt and pepper to taste
- ½ tsp paprika

Directions:
1. Add the beef into a skillet and cook over medium-high heat until it is browned completely.
2. Then, add in the minced garlic, stir, and cook for about 30 seconds.
3. Lower the heat to medium-low and add in the chili powder, paprika, cumin, oregano, and salt and pepper to taste. Stir to combine.
4. Now, pour the Rotel into the skillet, stir, and cover. Cook for 10 minutes.
5. Then, add the zucchini to the skillet, cover, and cook for an additional 10 minutes before serving.
6. Serve, and enjoy!

Hamburger Sausage and Broccoli Alfredo

Time: 50 minutes
Serving Size: 4 servings

Prep Time: 15 minutes

Cook Time: 35 minutes

Nutritional Facts/Info:

Calories 965

Carbs 8.3 g

Fat 65.7 g

Protein 81.8 g

Ingredients:
- 1 ½ lbs ground beef
- 1 lb ground sausage
- 1 tsp Italian seasoning
- 2 tsp minced garlic
- 6 oz cream cheese
- ½ medium onion chopped
- ⅓ cup Parmesan cheese grated
- ½ cup heavy whipping cream
- 1 cup mozzarella cheese shredded
- 3 cup broccoli florets
- salt and pepper to taste
- chopped parsley for garnish

Directions:
1. Preheat the oven to 350°F.
2. Put a large skillet over medium-high heat on the stove, and cook the ground beef, onions, and sausage until the meat is completely browned. Then, drain any extra fat.
3. As the meat browns, blanch the broccoli in boiling water for 5 minutes and then rinse and drain well with cold water.
4. Add some Italian seasoning, salt and pepper, and the minced garlic to the skillet, and stir to combine.
5. Reduce heat to medium-low. Place the cream cheese in the skillet, and stir until completely melted.
6. Now, add the Parmesan cheese and heavy whipping cream, and continue to cook for another few minutes.
7. Pour ⅔ of the meat mixture into the bottom of a 9" x 13" baking dish.
8. Top the meat mixture with some broccoli and then add the remaining ⅓ of the meat mixture.
9. Sprinkle the mozzarella cheese on top of the casserole, and bake for 25–30 minutes until browned and bubbly. Top with chopped parsley for garnish.
10. Serve, and enjoy!

Keto Cauliflower Pizza Crust

Time: 55 minutes
Serving Size: 1 serving

Prep Time: 15 minutes

Cook Time: 40 minutes

Nutritional Facts/Info:

Calories 69

Carbs 4 g

Fat 4 g

Protein 5 g

Ingredients:
- 2 cups riced cauliflower
- 1 large egg
- 1 tsp Italian seasoning
- ½ tsp garlic powder
- desired pizza sauce and toppings
- ⅔ cup Parmesan cheese, grated

Directions:
1. Preheat the oven to 400°F.
2. Rice the cauliflower in a food processor or blender.
3. Cook the cauliflower for 6 minutes in the microwave.

4. Add the cooked cauliflower rice and the other crust ingredients to a mixing bowl, and mix until combined.
5. Press the cauliflower dough into a thin circular shape on a parchment-lined baking sheet.
6. Bake for 15–20 minutes until a bit browned and cooked through.
7. Remove from the oven.
8. Add your favorite sauce and toppings, and then cook for an additional 10–15 minutes until browned to your liking.
9. Slice, serve, and enjoy!

Bacon Cheeseburger Soup

Time: 40 minutes
Serving Size: 1 serving

Prep Time: 15 minutes

Cook Time: 25 minutes

Nutritional Facts/Info:

Calories 624

Carbs 5 g

Fat 48 g

Protein 42 g

Ingredients:
- 1 ½ lb ground beef
- ½ cup bacon pieces
- 2 tbsp. butter
- 3 cups beef broth
- 2 tsp minced garlic
- 1 tsp Dijon mustard
- ½ tsp onion powder
- ½ medium onion, chopped
- 1 tsp chili powder
- ½ tsp cumin
- 2 tbsps Dill pickle relish
- 2 tbsps tomato paste

- 1 ¼ cup cheddar cheese, shredded
- 4 oz cream cheese
- salt and pepper to taste
- ½ cup heavy whipping cream

Directions:
1. Cook the meat alongside the onions in a deep skillet until the meat has turned completely brown and the onions have softened.
2. Add the butter, and all the spices to the meat, stirring to combine.
3. Meld together the wet ingredients (excluding the cream, cheddar cheese, and broth) and pour them into the skillet, mixing to incorporate the flavors.
4. Then add the broth and cheddar cheese, stirring frequently to melt the gooey cheese.
5. The heavy cream is added to thicken the soup, cook for several minutes until it reaches the thickness that you desire.
6. Serve topped with freshly chopped parsley, if desired.

Lasagna Stuffed Portobellos

Time: 50 minutes
Serving Size: 1 serving

Prep Time: 10 minutes

Cook Time: 40 minutes

Nutritional Facts/Info:

Calories 577

Carbs 11 g

Fat 46 g

Protein 31 g

Ingredients:
- 3 large Portobello mushroom caps
- ⅔ cup Ricotta
- ¾ lb Italian ground sausage
- ½ tsp Italian seasoning
- ¼ tsp garlic powder
- 1 cup mozzarella cheese shredded
- ½ cup marinara
- salt and pepper to taste
- chopped parsley for garnish

Directions:
1. Preheat the oven to 375°F.
2. Then, take 3 large Portobello mushroom cups and place them topside down in a dish of your choosing.
3. Create rough patty-like disks with the meat and press them into the mushroom cradles.
4. Place the ricotta, Italian seasoning, garlic powder, and the usual salt and pepper in a bowl, tossing to blend the flavors.
5. Top the meat mix by lathering on the ricotta mixture.
6. Finish the stuffed mushrooms with a dollop of marinara sauce and the shredded cheese.
7. Bake the mushrooms for 35–40 minutes.
8. Allow them to cool, and top them with some freshly chopped parsley.
9. Serve, and enjoy!

Pesto Spinach Artichoke Chicken Bake

Time: 55 minutes
Serving Size: 1 serving

Prep Time: 15 minutes

Cook Time: 40 minutes

Nutritional Facts/Info:

Calories 1016

Carbs 45.9 g

Fat 68.8 g

Protein 53.9 g

Ingredients:
- ¼ cup Pesto sauce
- 2 large boneless skinless chicken breasts
- 2 small tomatoes chopped
- 2-3 cup raw spinach
- ¼ cup parmesan cheese, grated
- 1 cup marinated artichoke hearts
- salt and pepper to taste if desired
- 1 ½ cup mozzarella cheese

Directions:
1. Preheat the oven to 375°F.
2. Slice the chicken breasts in half lengthwise to form four servings of chicken.
3. Place the chicken in a single layer at the bottom of a baking dish. You can add salt and pepper to taste if desired.
4. Spread the pesto sauce evenly over the chicken pieces.
5. Place some spinach, marinated artichoke hearts, and tomatoes on top of the chicken.
6. Now sprinkle the Parmesan cheese over the casserole.
7. Then, top the mixture with the mozzarella cheese.
8. Bake for 35–40 minutes in the oven until the chicken is cooked through.
9. Serve, and enjoy!

Bacon Ranch Chicken Crust Pizza

Time: 55 minutes
Serving Size: 8 servings

Prep Time: 15 minutes

Cook Time: 40 minutes

Nutritional Facts/Info:

Calories 291

Carbs 1.5 g

Fat 17.1 g

Protein 28.7 g

Ingredients:
For the crust:
- 1 lb ground chicken
- ⅓ cup mozzarella cheese shredded
- ½ cup Parmesan cheese grated
- ½ tsp oregano
- 1 egg
- salt and pepper to taste.
- ½ tsp basil

For the sauce:
- ¼ cup sour cream
- 1 tbsp ranch seasoning mix

- 3 oz cream cheese softened
- 2 tbsp freshly chopped chives

Toppings:
- 1 ½ cup mozzarella cheese
- ½ medium tomato chopped
- ½ cup chopped bacon pieces

Directions:
1. Preheat the oven to 400°F.
2. Add the ingredients meant for the crust into a large mixing bowl, and combine well.
3. Spread the mixture for the crust onto a parchment-lined baking sheet, and create circles by molding it with your hands. Make the crust as thin or thick as you desire.
4. It should take 35–40 minutes to bake, but check that the meat has fully cooked and the crust has crisped to a golden brown.
5. Now, mix the ingredients for the sauce.
6. Then, cover the top of the pizza with the sauce mixture.
7. Add the tomato, mozzarella cheese, and bacon pieces on top of the sauce.
8. Let the cheese melt in the oven for another 10 minutes.
9. Slice, serve, and enjoy!

Moroccan Meatballs

Time: 1 hour 15 minutes
Serving Size: 12 meatballs

Prep Time: 15 minutes

Cook Time: 1 hour

Nutritional Facts/Info:

Calories 164

Carbs 2.9 g

Fat 6.8 g

Protein 22 g

Ingredients:
Meatballs Ingredients
- 2 lbs ground lamb
- ½ cup fresh parsley leaves, minced
- 1 tsp paprika
- 2 tsp ground cumin
- 1 tsp salt
- ¼ tsp ground black pepper

Sauce Ingredients
- 3 medium tomatoes, diced
- ½ cup tomato juice
- ½ cup fresh parsley leaves, minced

- 1 tbsp coconut oil
- 2 medium onions, diced
- 2 garlic cloves, crushed
- 2 tsp paprika
- 2 tsp ground cumin
- 1 tsp salt
- ¼ tsp ground black pepper
- 1 ½ cups water

Directions:
1. Use a large bowl to combine the parsley, paprika, cumin, salt, and pepper.
2. Now use your hands to crumble the lamb into the bowl and knead all of the ingredients together.
3. Wet your hands with some water, then take about a tablespoon of the lamb and roll it into a ball between your palms.
4. Place it on a baking sheet. Continue to roll the entire mixture of lamb until all of the meat is formed into balls and lined up on the baking sheet.
5. Heat the oil in a large pot on medium heat.
6. Add the onion and sauté until soft and translucent.
7. Now add to the pot the garlic, paprika, cumin, salt, and pepper and stir for a minute or two.
8. Add the chopped tomatoes, tomato juice, parsley, and water, and stir. Bring the sauce to a boil.
9. Gently drop the meatballs into the sauce, cover, and reduce heat to simmer.
10. Cook, covered, for 40 minutes, then remove the cover and cook an additional 20 minutes.
11. Serve, and enjoy!

Keto Tacos

Time: 1 hour
Serving Size: 8 tacos

Prep Time: 30 minutes

Cook Time: 30 minutes

Nutritional Facts/Info:

Calories 261

Carbs 2 g

Fat 21 g

Protein 17 g

Ingredients:
- 1 lb ground beef
- 2 tbsps homemade taco seasoning
- 1/4 cup water

Toppings for a taco:
- sour cream
- avocado
- cheese
- lettuce

Directions:
1. Preheat the oven to 350°F.
2. On a baking sheet lined with parchment paper or a silicone placemat.
3. Place 1/4 cup piles of cheese 2 inches apart. Press the cheese down lightly so it makes one layer.
4. Place baking sheet in the oven and bake for 5–7 minutes or until the edges of the cheese are brown.
5. Let the cheese cool for 1–2 minutes until it is firm enough to lift but still bendable. Lift the cheese and place it over the handle of a spoon or other utensil that is balanced on two cups.
6. Let the cheese cool completely then remove.
7. While you continue to bake your cheese taco shells place the ground beef in a skillet over medium-high heat cooking until it is completely cooked through.
8. Drain the grease from the meat and then add the homemade taco seasoning. Pour water into the skillet and stir everything around mixing it.
9. Simmer for 5 minutes or until liquid has cooked away.
10. Add meat to taco shells and top with your favorite taco toppings

Low Carb Big Mac Bites

Time: 35 minutes
Serving Size: 16 servings

Prep Time: 20 minutes

Cook Time: 15 minutes

Nutritional Facts/Info:

Calories 182

Carbs 1 g

Fat 12 g

Protein 10 g

Ingredients:
- ¼ cup onion, finely diced
- 1.5 lbs ground beef
- 4 slices American cheese
- 1 tsp salt
- lettuce
- 16 slices Dill pickle

Secret Sauce
- 1/2 cup mayonnaise
- 2 tbsps yellow mustard
- 4 tbsps Dill pickle relish
- 1 tsp paprika

- 1 tsp white wine vinegar
- 1 tsp garlic powder
- 1 tsp onion powder

Directions:

11. Preheat the oven to 400°F.
12. Use a large bowl to combine the onions, ground beef, and salt. Mix until thoroughly combined, you can use your hands.
13. Wet your hands with water and then roll the beef into 1.5-ounce balls. Create mini burger patties by flattening them gently with your hand making sure not to let them crumble before gently placing them on a baking tray.
14. Bake at 400°F for 15 minutes or until cooked through.
15. As the burgers cook, meld together the secret sauce ingredients in a bowl by stirring well.
16. Remove the burgers when the meaty smells waft through the whole house. Then, pat any excess grease off.
17. Quickly cube the cheese slices and place a square on each patty popping them back in the oven (which should be turned off at this point) to let the cheese melt and ooze down the sides.
18. Assemble the skewers by adding a square of lettuce, a slice of pickle, and the cooked meat to the skewer sticks.
19. Serve with the secret sauce and enjoy!

Keto Fried Chicken in the Air Fryer

Time: 40 minutes
Serving Size: 8 servings

Prep Time: 20 minutes

Cook Time: 20 minutes

Nutritional Facts/Info:

Calories 151

Carbs 4 g

Fat 11 g

Protein 10 g

Ingredients:
- 2 lbs chicken, breasts, thighs, and legs
- 1 cup almond flour
- 1 tsp salt
- 2.5 oz crushed pork rinds
- 2 tsp garlic powder
- 2 tsp onion powder
- 1 tsp black pepper
- 2 tsp paprika
- 3 tbsps water
- cooking spray
- 2 large eggs

Directions:
1. Combine the crushed pork rinds, onion powder, paprika, almond flour, salt, garlic powder, and pepper and pour into a shallow bowl or on a large plate.
2. Crack the eggs into a second bowl and add the water. Then whisk till you get consistency.
3. Coat each piece of chicken by first dipping it in the egg mixture, then rolling it in the almond flour mixture to coat it. You can use your hands to make sure the flour coats the chicken completely.
4. Set aside each coated chicken piece.
5. Once all of the pieces of chicken are breaded, preheat your air fryer to 350°F.
6. Then, lightly spray 2 pieces of chicken with cooking spray and place them in the basket of your air fryer.
7. Cook for 9 minutes, then open the air fryer, gently turn the chicken over, and place the basket back in the fryer to continue cooking for 9 minutes more.
8. Take the pieces out of the air fryer.
9. Serve and enjoy.

Keto Easy Herb-Roasted Turkey

Time: 4 hrs 15 mins
Serving Size: 1 turkey

Prep Time: 15 mins

Cook Time: 3 hrs 30 mins

Nutritional Facts/Info:

Calories 597

Carbs 0.9 g

Fat 33.7 g

Protein 68.2 g

Ingredients:
- ¾ cup olive oil
- 1 (12 lbs) whole turkey
- 2 tsp dried basil
- 2 tbsps garlic powder
- 1 tsp salt
- 1 tsp ground sage
- 2 cups water
- ½ tsp black pepper

Directions:
1. Preheat the oven to 325°F.
2. Clean the turkey (discard giblets and organs), and place it in a roasting pan with a lid.
3. Use a small bowl to combine olive oil, dried basil, ground sage, garlic powder, salt, and black pepper.
4. Using a brush, baste the entire uncooked turkey with sauce with a brush.
5. Create a pool of water at the bottom of the roasting pan before covering.
6. Once baking the inside of the thickest part of the turkey thigh should reach 180°F, this will take 3 or 3 ½ hours.
7. Remove the bird from the oven, and allow it to stand for about 30 minutes before carving.
8. Serve, and enjoy!

Pork Fried Rice

Time: 30 minutes
Serving Size: 4 servings

Prep Time: 15 minutes

Cook Time: 15 minutes

Nutritional Facts/Info:

Calories 943

Carbs 162.9 g

Fat 15 g

Protein 34.5 g

Ingredients:
- 2 tbsp. vegetable oil, divided
- 3 large eggs, lightly beaten
- 1/2 onion, chopped
- 1 carrot, peeled and cut into 1/4" pieces
- 200 g minced pork
- Salt
- freshly ground black pepper
- 1 tbsp grated ginger
- 2 cloves garlic, crushed
- 150 g frozen peas
- 750 g cooked white rice
- 2 tbsp low-sodium soy sauce

- 1 tbsp hoisin sauce
- 3 spring onions, thinly sliced
- 1 tsp sesame oil

Directions:
1. Put a large skillet over medium heat, and heat 1 tablespoon vegetable oil.
2. Add the eggs and let them sit for a few seconds before lightly scrambling and folding the egg mixture over itself.
3. Then, remove them from the skillet and set them aside.
4. Use the same skillet to heat the remaining tablespoon of oil, and add onion and carrot.
5. Cook, stirring occasionally until the vegetables are tender.
6. Now add the ground pork to the skillet and season with salt and pepper (if desired)
7. Then cook until the pork is no longer pink and is starting to caramelize.
8. Stir in the ginger, garlic, and peas, and cook until fragrant.
9. Now add the rice and stir in the soy sauce, hoisin, spring onions, and sesame oil.
10. Toss to combine then fold in scrambled eggs.
11. Serve immediately, and enjoy!

Roast Pork Belly

Time: 1 hour 30 minutes
Serving Size: 4 servings

Prep Time: 30 minutes

Cook Time: 1 hour

Nutritional Facts/Info:

Calories 3911

Carbs 71.2 g

Fat 367.7 g

Protein 69.4 g

Ingredients:
- 4 lb piece boneless pork belly
- 1 bulb fennel, quartered
- 2 carrots, roughly chopped
- 2 sticks celery, roughly chopped
- 1 bulb garlic, halved
- 2 medium onions, quartered
- 1 bunch thyme
- 5-star anise
- 2 tsp fennel seeds
- 1 tsp black peppercorns
- 6 tsp flaky sea salt
- 1 bottle of white wine

- 50 g flour
- 50 ml vegetable oil

Directions:
1. Pre-heat oven to 240°F.
2. Rub oil over the skin of the pork. With a pestle and mortar, crush fennel seeds and salt and rub liberally all over the pork joint.
3. In a large roasting tin, place fennel, onions, carrots, and celery to form a trivet that the pork will sit on. Add garlic, thyme, star anise, black peppercorns, and remaining oil. Toss together.
4. Lay pork belly over the vegetables and cook in the oven for 30 minutes or until the crackling starts to crisp up.
5. Turn the oven down to 374°F and add half the bottle of wine to the roasting tray. Cook for a further 60–90min.
6. After this, add the rest of the wine to the tray and cook for a further hour. The meat should be soft and tender. If the skin is not as crisp as required turn the oven temp back up to 474°F for the remaining 15 minutes of cooking.
7. Remove pork belly, cover with foil and allow to rest while you make gravy.
8. To make gravy, put roasting tin with all leftover juices over hob on medium heat. Add flour and stir, allowing the juices to cookout and thicken for a minute. Add a little water to thickened pan juices, and bring to a slow boil until it turns into a sauce consistency. Pass the sauce through a sieve to remove any lump and leftover veggies, and check to season.
9. Slice pork into six equal pieces, and serve alongside gravy with mash and your choice of vegetables.

Keto Cheeseburger Sushi

Time: 50 minutes
Serving Size: 4 servings

Prep Time: 10 minutes

Cook Time: 40 minutes

Nutritional Facts/Info:

Calories 602

Carbs 3.45 g

Fat 50.8 g

Protein 30.7 g

Ingredients:
- 16-ounce ground beef
- salt and pepper to taste
- 10 slice bacon
- 2 oz cheddar cheese
- 2 medium dill pickles, diced
- 1/2 medium red onion, sliced
- 2 tbsps low-carb ketchup
- 1/4 cup mayonnaise
- 2 tsp unsweetened dill pickle relish
- 1 tbsp yellow mustard

Directions:
1. Get all the ingredients ready.
2. Preheat the oven to 375°F.
3. Take a piece of plastic wrap, and layer the bacon slices on top of each other.
4. Then, spread the ground beef on top of the bacon. Make sure that you spread it out thin to ensure that it fully cooks. Season with salt and pepper (if desired).
5. Now, place the cheddar cheese, sliced dill pickles, and sliced red onion on the half of the ground beef that is closest to you. Stop the topping with a clean line to make it easier to roll properly.
6. Tightly enclose the fillings by carefully rolling the bacon, enclosing everything inside, toothpicks are necessary to help keep the roll tucked in while cooking.
7. Place the roll on a baking sheet and bake for 40 minutes or until fully cooked through.
8. Instead of drooling over the cooking cheeseburger sushi, rather keep busy by making the dipping sauce. Start by combining mayonnaise, ketchup, yellow mustard, and dill pickle relish in a bowl. Stir this together until it is fully incorporated, then leave it for later use.
9. Hold on while it cools, before cutting the 'sushi' into rolls, one per serving.
10. Serve, and enjoy!

Keto Chicken and Broccoli Wok Meal

Time: 30 minutes
Serving Size: 4 servings

Prep Time: 15 minutes

Cook Time: 15 minutes

Nutritional Facts/Info:

Calories 552

Carbs 10.7 g

Fat 44.1 g

Protein 27.4 g

Ingredients:
- 2 tbsps coconut oil
- 1/2 medium onion
- 8 oz broccoli
- salt and pepper to taste
- 8 oz green cabbage, thinly sliced
- 12 oz canned coconut milk
- 12 oz cooked chicken
- 2 tbsps peanut butter
- 1.5 tbsp green curry paste
- 2 tbsp green onion, for garnish
- 1 oz peanuts, for garnish

Directions:
1. Prepare all the ingredients.
2. You need cooked chicken for this recipe. If you do not have it, you can sauté boneless, skinless chicken thighs until cooked through.
3. Peel and cut the onion into wedges. Slice up the cabbage finely. Keep the florets and stems of the broccoli in one piece by cutting the vegetable lengthways.
4. Drop a dash of the coconut oil into the wok.
5. Heat on medium to high heat, then toss in the cut-up onion, broccoli, and sliced cabbage, shaking the pan to mix well before seasoning with salt and pepper to taste (if desired).
6. Cube the cooked chicken into bite-sized pieces before shaking them into the pan along with the coconut milk, peanut butter, and green curry paste. Shake the pan until the ingredients sizzle together and the flavors begin to blend into each other.
7. Let the dish begin to simmer for 2–5 minutes allowing the flavors to seep in. Season again according to your spice preference.
8. Garnish with peanuts and green onions.
9. Serve, and enjoy!

Chapter 6: Keto Snacks

Starting a diet is simpler than staying on it. Being on the go and visiting friends or relatives can throw you off the wagon. Not to mention those sugar cravings that promise to get you to cheat on your diet. This is where snacks come in. When you have good snacking meals, you can survive sugar cravings and avoid eating things that you shouldn't when on the go.

Oven-Baked Bacon Chips

Time: 25 minutes
Serving Size: 15 servings

Prep Time: 5 minutes

Cook Time: 20 minutes

Nutritional Facts/Info:

Calories 103

Carbs 0.3 g

Fat 2.6 g

Protein 7 g

Ingredients:
- 1 package thick-cut bacon

Directions:
1. Preheat the oven to 400°F.
2. Get a baking dish and line it with the non-stick paper of your choice. Parchment paper will do, but if you prefer, a silicone baking mat works wonders.
3. Using scissors, cut up the bacon into 2-inch squares.
4. Use the bacon squares as a base and add the chips on top of the squares, and make sure that you leave small spaces between the pieces so that they do not stick together.
5. Bake the chips for 20 minutes. If your bacon is thinly cut, bake the pieces for 15 minutes. Adding more time adds crisper to the chip and we all love a little crisp, don't we?
6. Let cool for 10 minutes on the tray before transferring to a plate.
7. Serve alone or with guacamole and ENJOY!

Keto Guacamole

Time: 15 minutes
Serving Size: 1 serving

Prep Time: 15 minutes

Nutritional Facts/Info:

Calories 938 | Carbs 30.8 g | Fat 15.3 g |Protein 5.5 g

Ingredients:
- 1 large avocado, peeled and pitted (approximately 6 ounces)
- grated zest of 1 lime
- juice of 1 Lime
- 1/2 tsp finely ground salt
- 1 tbsp with an additional 1 teaspoon apple cider vinegar
- 2 tsp fresh chives, sliced
- 1 tbsp plus 1 tsp dried oregano leaves
- 2 tbsp fresh cilantro, finely chopped
- 1/4 cup with an additional 2 tbsp MCT oil
- 1/2 tsp ground black pepper

Directions:
1. Place the avocado, dried oregano, vinegar, oil, lime zest and juice, salt, and pepper in a large bowl.
2. Then, mash everything with a potato masher. Forks work just as well if you don't have a masher. Mash until smooth and creamy unless you prefer your guacamole to be left slightly chunky.
3. Stir in the fresh cilantro and chives.
4. Serve, and enjoy!

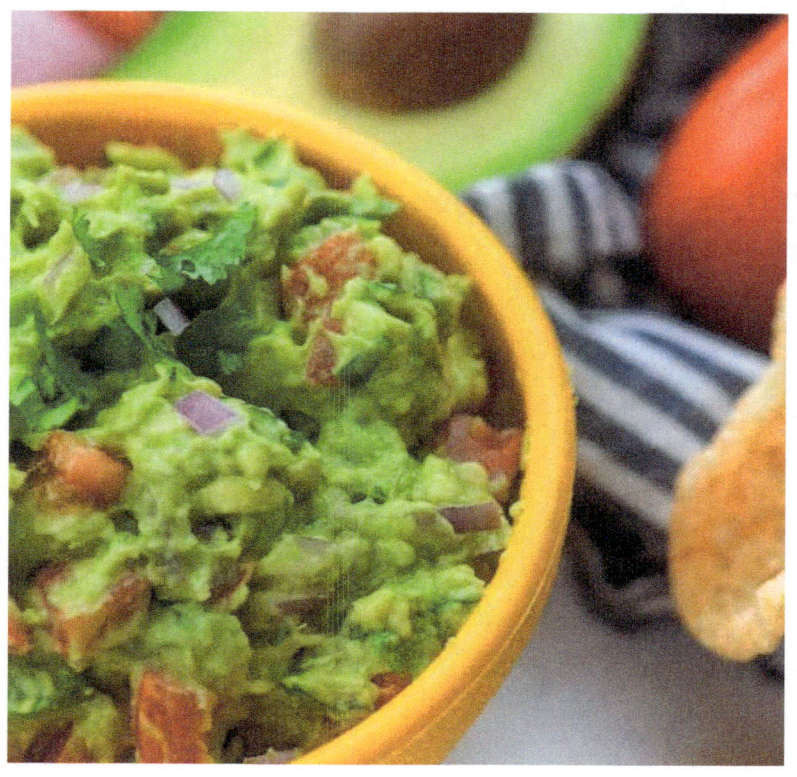

Caramel Glazed Keto Donut Holes

Who said donuts can't go low carb? These donut holes are a must-have for pastry lovers.
Time: 25 minutes
Serving Size: 12 donut holes

Prep Time: 10 minutes

Cook Time: 15 minutes

Nutritional Facts/Info:

Calories 165 | Carbs 8 g | Fat 14 g | Protein 5 g

Ingredients:
Donut Holes
- 1 cup water
- 2 tbsp butter unsalted
- 1 tsp baking powder
- 3/4 cup coconut flour
- 2 tbsp monk fruit
- 1 cup almond flour
- 1 egg

Caramel Topping
- 3 tbsp butter unsalted, softened
- ¼ cup natural almond butter
- 2 tsp cinnamon
- 2 tbsp monk fruit

Directions:

Donut Holes Instructions
1. Preheat the oven to 375°F.
2. In the meantime, line a baking sheet with a baking mat, such as a silicone mat or, if you only have parchment paper on hand, that will do, too.
3. Bring a mix of butter and water to boiling point in a medium-sized saucepan. Then, take it off the stove, letting the bubbles fade as it cools down for 3 minutes.
4. Toss the dry ingredients (almond flour, monk fruit, coconut flour, and baking powder) in the bowl to create a powdered mix.
5. Add the water/butter mixture and the egg to the powdered mix and whisk them up, forming a complex dough that holds together but is soft to the touch.
6. Roll up the springy doll, creating the fluffiness of the soon-to-be donut by rubbing oil into small 2-inch balls.
7. Place the donuts on the tray and bake for 15 minutes or until their exteriors turn a subtle brown.
8. Then, remove from the oven to cool while you whip up the mouth-watering caramel topping.

Caramel Topping Instructions

9. Whisk the monk fruit and cinnamon together, and set aside.
10. Use a separate bowl, whisk together the almond butter and softened butter until both kinds of butter are uniform in color as they become one. Add the contents of the dry mix bowl, stir until well combined.
11. Coat the donuts in the sauce by rolling them around. Being sure to cover every inch with that delicious caramel sauce—you wouldn't want to miss a spot.
12. Allow drying.

Keto Fudge Brownies

These almond flour fudge brownies are oh so delicious, and they promise to satisfy your cravings.
Time: 25 minutes
Serving Size: 16 brownies

Prep Time: 10 minutes

Cook Time: 15 minutes

Nutritional Facts/Info:

Calories 174

Carbs 4 g

Fat 16 g

Protein 3 g

Ingredients:
- 1/2 cup butter
- 1/4 cup walnuts (optional)
- 1 tsp vanilla extract (optional)
- 2/3 cup Best Powdered Allulose (or powdered erythritol)
- 2 tbsp cocoa powder
- 3/4 cup Wholesome Yum Blanched Almond Flour
- 2 large eggs (at room temperature)
- 4 oz unsweetened baking chocolate
- 1/4 tsp sea salt (only if using unsalted butter)

Directions:
1. Preheat the oven to 350°F.
2. Fully cover an 8" x 8" inch pan using a large piece of parchment paper, allowing the paper to fold over the sides of the pan.
3. Watching the chocolate melt is the best part. Combine it with the butter in a double boiler, allowing them to reach a smooth sauce, incorporating them with a spoon. Move them away from the heat once melted.
4. Add in the vanilla extract.
5. Add the almond flour, cocoa powder, powdered sweetener, eggs, and sea salt. Stir together until everything is completely combined. The batter will be a little grainy looking.
6. Transfer the batter to the lined pan. Then, smooth the top with something flat such as a spatula or the backside of a spoon. Press some chopped walnuts into the doughy parcels.
7. The wait is not too long with only about 13–18 minutes of baking. You'll know it's ready when the dough has amalgamated together. Poke it with a toothpick and, if it comes out clean or with some firm batter, it's gone time.
8. Cool completely before moving or cutting. If there is butter pooled on top, leave it (it will be absorbed after cooling).
9. Serve, and enjoy!

Grain-Free Amaretto Cookies

Time: 30 minutes
Serving Size: 16 cookies

Prep Time: 10 minutes

Cook Time: 20 minutes

Nutritional Facts/Info:

Calories 71

Carbs 7.1 g

Fat 5.9 g

Protein 2.5 g

Ingredients:
- 2 cups almond meal
- 1/4 cup granular erythritol
- 2 tsp baking powder
- 1/2 tsp almond extract
- 1/4 cup unsweetened applesauce
- 1/2 cup powdered erythritol (to shake)
- 1/4 tsp pure Madagascar Bourbon Vanilla Extract
- 1/4 tsp cinnamon

Directions:
1. Preheat the oven to 350°F.
2. Use a large mixing bowl to combine and mix all ingredients (not the powdered erythritol) to form your cookie dough.
3. Roll 16 (1 tablespoon each) balls and place them in a plastic bag with the powdered erythritol. Shake the plastic bag to coat the balls.
4. Prepare a baking sheet with parchment paper and space the powdered dough balls out evenly.
5. Then, press the balls down a bit with your fingers to flatten them.
6. Bake for 20 minutes in the heated oven, remove and let cool.
7. Store in an airtight container.
8. Serve, and enjoy!

Low-Carb Cheese Crackers

Time: 30 minutes
Serving Size: 30 servings

Prep Time: 10 minutes

Cook Time: 20 minutes

Nutritional Facts/Info:

Calories 123

Carbs 2 g

Fat 10.2 g

Protein 6 g

Ingredients:
- 1 cup almond flour
- 2 oz cream cheese
- 1 egg
- 2 cups cheese of your choice
- 1/2 tsp sea salt
- 1 tsp rosemary

Directions:
1. Create a cheesy delight by combining them all (including the cream cheese) along with the almond flour in a microwave-safe bowl and set the cooking time to 1 minute. If you prefer not to use the microwave, feel free to use a stovetop.
2. Before the cheese sets, quickly mix in the flour; you only want the cheese slightly melted, but not hard either.
3. Let them settle into each other for a few minutes, cooling down enough to not cook the egg when added.
4. At a reasonable temperature, add the egg, pinch of salt, and any seasoning that gets your taste buds tingling. A teaspoon will be sufficient or be generous if you prefer.
5. Evenly distribute these added spices by mixing well and if your fork is getting stuck, the cheese has hardened. A quick burst in the microwave will soften it up enough to continue mixing.
6. Now you get to play with a cheesy ball—what a dream! Roll it around using parchment paper, a rolling pin, or my favorite tool ever, hands, to spread it into a thin cheesy layer.
7. You have more options here to either use a cookie cutter or a pizza knife to square the cracker batter into the size you desire.
8. Each side should be baked for about 5 to 6 minutes at a heat of 450°F. Use the parchment paper (it won't be as hot as the crackers) to flip them to bake the other side. Bake until you spot the crispy level.
9. Don't burn your mouth! Let them cool for 5 minutes, while the flavors settle before munching away.

Keto Sugar-Free Chocolate Pudding

Time: 5 minutes
Serving Size: 4 servings

Prep Time: 5 minutes

Cook Time: 10 minutes

Nutritional Facts/Info:

Calories 431

Carbs 6 g

Fat 43 g

Protein 5 g

Ingredients:
- 2 cups heavy cream (divided into 1/4 cup and 1 3/4 cup)
- 2 tsp vanilla extract
- 1/3 cup Best Powdered Erythritol
- 1/4 tsp sea salt
- 1/4 cup cocoa powder
- 1 1/2 tsp unflavored gelatin powder

Directions:
1. Take a small bowl and pour 1/4 cup heavy cream.
2. Sprinkle the gelatin powder on top, and whisk together immediately. Set aside.
3. In a medium saucepan over medium-low heat, stir together the remaining heavy cream, cocoa powder, powdered sweetener, and sea salt.
4. Heat the mixture, whisking constantly, for 5 minutes, until the mixture is smooth and bubbling near the edges.
5. Remove from heat. Then, stir in the vanilla extract.
6. Add the gelatin to the pan and whisk until smooth and dissolved.
7. Now, let the pudding cool for about 10 minutes, until cooled enough not to melt the plastic wrap over it. Whisk again to get rid of any film on top.
8. Cover with plastic wrap flush against the top to prevent a film from forming. Refrigerate for at least 2 hours, until firm.
9. Serve, and enjoy!

Keto Low Carb Lemon Blueberry Bread

Time: 45 minutes
Serving Size: 10 servings

Prep Time: 15 minutes

Cook Time: 30 minutes

Nutritional Facts/Info:

Calories 267

Carbs 7 g

Fat 25 g

Protein 6 g

Ingredients:
- 2 cups almond flour
- 2 tsp baking powder
- lemon zest from 1/4–1/2 lemon
- 2 eggs
- 1/2–1 cup blueberry
- 1/2 cup erythritol
- 1 tbsp lemon juice
- 1/4 cup butter, melted
- 1 cup heavy whipping cream

Directions:
1. Preheat the oven to 350°F.
2. Use a mixing bowl to combine the eggs, melted butter, and heavy whipping cream that has been cooled a bit. Then beat for several minutes until everything is combined.
3. Use a separate mixing bowl to add together the almond flour, baking powder, erythritol, and lemon zest. Then mix to combine.
4. Now, add the dry ingredients to the wet ingredients, and beat until just combined.
5. Pour in 1 tbsp of lemon juice and stir. Then, fold in the blueberries.
6. Pour the mixture into a greased loaf pan, then bake for 30–45 minutes until a knife inserted into the center of the bread comes out clean.
7. Let cool,
8. Slice, serve, and enjoy immediately or store in the fridge in an airtight container.

Healthy Avocado Chocolate Cookies

Time: 15 minutes
Serving Size: 15 cookies

Prep Time: 5 minutes

Cook Time: 10 minutes

Nutritional Facts/Info:

Calories 115

Carbs 13 g

Fat 7 g

Protein 2 g

Ingredients:
- 2 avocados peeled, pit removed
- 1/2 cup cocoa powder unsweetened
- 1/4 cup almond flour
- 2 eggs
- 1/2 cup coconut sugar
- 1/2 cup chocolate chips
- 1/2 tsp baking soda

Directions:
1. Preheat the oven to 350°F.
2. Add all the ingredients (except chocolate chips) to a food processor and blend until smooth.
3. Stir in the chocolate chips by hand.
4. Spoon onto a baking pan covered with a sheet of lightly greased foil, or non-stick silicone baking mat.
5. Bake for 10 minutes at 350°F.
6. Remove from oven and allow to cool to room temperature
7. Then store in an airtight container in the fridge (for 2–3 days) or freezer (for about a week)
8. Serve, and enjoy!

Keto Fermented Dill Pickles

Time: 3 days 10 minutes
Serving Size: 4 jars

Prep Time: 10 minutes

Cook Time: 3 days

Nutritional Facts/Info:

Calories 53

Carbs 9 g

Fat 0 g

Protein 3 g

Ingredients:
- 1 kg (2 lbs) of mini cucumbers
- 2 l water
- 1.5 tbsp colorful peppercorns
- 1 tbsp cloves
- 4 tbsp salt
- 8 dry bay leaves
- dill
- 1.5 tbsp mustard seeds
- 4 garlic cloves
- 4 grape leaves
- 1 parsnip
- 1 carrot

- 4 chili peppers
- 1 ginger

Directions:
1. Scrub the vegetables with water and focus on cleaning those cucumbers well. Then spread them on a kitchen cloth to allow them to fully dry.
2. Boil some water, and add some salt. Once the water starts bubbling, add the salt and watch that it dissolves. Then, switch the water off and let it cool fully.
3. Add the colorful peppercorn, mustard seeds, and then cloves into the cooled water. Mix everything and set it aside.
4. Get your mason jars ready for action, or any other type of jar you have.
5. First, place the dill leaves at the bottom of each jar.
6. Cut the veggies (except cucumbers) into slices. Arrange the slices (use the colors well to create colorful layers) inside the jars over the bed of dill leaves.
7. Start by adding a few cucumbers into each mason jar.
8. Then add one wine leaf on the side of the jar. This special touch will pull the flavors of the fermented dill pickles together.
9. Put more veggies, such as ginger, dill, and cucumbers, into the mason jar.
10. Once the jar is filled to about 3/4, add a touch of spice by popping in one red chili pepper to each jar.
11. Complete the finishing touch by placing cucumbers on top of the pickled array.
12. The spice-infused water should then be poured in, allowing it to trickle down to the bottom of the jar.
13. Stop pouring right before the jar overflows, eliminating any chance of air spoiling the pickled jars.
14. Leave the jars to ferment for 3 days.

Buffalo Cauliflower Bites

Time: 40 minutes
Serving Size: 6 servings

Prep Time: 10 minutes

Cook Time: 30 minutes

Nutritional Facts/Info:

Calories 209

Carbs 6.4 g

Fat 19.5 g

Protein 5.9 g

Ingredients:
- 1 cup almond meal
- 1 tsp granulated garlic
- 1/2 tsp dried parsley
- 1/2 tsp salt
- 1 large egg
- 1 large head cauliflower, cut into bite-sized florets
- 1/2 cup Frank's RedHot sauce
- 1/4 cup ghee

Directions:
1. Preheat the oven to 400°F.
2. Line a baking sheet with a baking mat or paper.
3. Combine the almond meal, parsley, garlic, and salt in a large sealable plastic bag and shake to mix.
4. Use a large bowl to whisk the egg and add cauliflower and toss to coat completely.
5. Transfer the cauliflower to a bag filled with almond meal mixture and toss to coat.
6. Arrange cauliflower in a single layer on a baking sheet ready to bake away for 30 minutes, or until softened and slightly browned.
7. While cauliflower is baking, combine hot sauce and ghee in a small saucepan over low heat.
8. When the cauliflower is cooked, combine cauliflower with hot sauce mixture in a large mixing bowl and toss to coat.
9. Serve, and enjoy!

Keto Crackers

Time: 22 minutes
Serving Size: 6 servings

Prep Time: 10 minutes

Cook Time: 12 minutes

Nutritional Facts/Info:

Calories 298

Carbs 7.5 g

Fat 22.3 g

Protein 15.0 g

Ingredients:
- 1 cup grated Parmesan cheese
- 1 cup shredded cheddar cheese
- 2 oz (¼ cup) cream cheese, softened
- 1 cup almond flour
- 1 large egg, lightly beaten
- ½ tsp salt
- 1 tsp granulated garlic
- ½ tsp dried rosemary

Directions:
1. Preheat the oven to 450°F.
2. Then cover up a baking tray using parchment paper and combine the Parmesan, cheddar, and cream cheeses, along with the almond flour, in a medium saucepan over low heat.
3. Keep stirring the cheese until melted.
4. Then, remove from heat and allow to cool.
5. Once the cheese mixture has cooled enough, add the egg and spices and stir to combine. The mixture should look dough-like.
6. Cradle the dough in the middle of two pieces of parchment paper and roll out into a rectangle.
7. Cut the dough into crackers, approximately 1½" squares, and arrange in a single layer on the baking sheet.
8. Bake for 12 minutes, turning crackers over once during cooking. If, after 12 minutes, the crackers are still not crispy, continue baking until they reach your desired level of crispness.
9. Allow cooling slightly before eating.
10. Serve, and enjoy!

Garlic and Bacon Dip

Time: 45 minutes
Serving Size: 6 servings

Prep Time: 15 minutes

Cook Time: 30 minutes

Nutritional Facts/Info:

Calories 271

Carbs 5.3 g

Fat 20.4 g

Protein 11.4 g

Ingredients:
- 8 slices no-sugar-added bacon
- 2 cups chopped spinach
- 1 (8-oz) package cream cheese, softened
- 1/4 cup full-fat sour cream
- 1/4 cup plain full-fat Greek yogurt
- 2 tbsps chopped fresh parsley
- 1 tbsp lemon juice
- 6 cloves roasted garlic, mashed
- 1 tsp salt
- 1/2 tsp black pepper
- 1/2 cup grated Parmesan cheese

Directions:
1. Preheat the oven to 350°F.
2. Cook the bacon in a medium skillet over medium heat until crispy.
3. Remove the bacon from the pan and we don't want them too greasy so use some paper towels and get rid of that excess oil.
4. Add spinach to a hot pan and cook until wilted. Then remove it from the heat and set it aside.
5. Add cream cheese, sour cream, yogurt, lemon juice, garlic, parsley, salt, and pepper and beat with a handheld mixer until combined.
6. Roughly chop bacon and stir into cream cheese mixture. Stir in spinach and Parmesan cheese.
7. Transfer to an 8" × 8" baking pan and bake for 30 minutes or until steaming hot and gently bubbling.
8. Once cooked, serve, and enjoy!

Chicken Skin Crisps with Spicy Avocado Cream (Fat Bombs)

Time: 25 minutes
Serving Size: 6 fat bombs

Prep Time: 10 minutes

Cook Time: 15 minutes

Nutritional Facts/Info:

Calories 86

Carbs 0.7 g

Fat 7.5 g

Protein 2.6 g

Ingredients:
- Skin from 3 large chicken thighs
- ¼ medium avocado, peeled and pitted
- 3 tbsps full-fat sour cream
- ½ medium jalapeño pepper, seeded and finely chopped
- ½ tsp sea salt

Directions:
1. Preheat the oven to 350°F.
2. On a baking sheet lined with parchment paper layout skins as flat as possible.
3. Bake for 12–15 minutes until the skins turn light brown and crispy, be careful not to burn them.
4. Remove skins from the baking sheet and place them on a paper towel to cool and allow the excess grease to drain.
5. In a small bowl, combine avocado, sour cream, jalapeño, and salt.
6. Mix everything with a fork until well combined.
7. Cut each crispy chicken skin into 2 pieces.
8. Place 1 tablespoon avocado mix on each chicken crisp and serve immediately.
9. Enjoy!

Cheesy Meatballs

Time: 40 minutes
Serving Size: 4 servings

Prep Time: 10 minutes

Cook Time: 30 minutes

Nutritional Facts/Info:

Calories 668

Carbs 3.2 g

Fat 40.8 g

Protein 70.1 g

Ingredients:
- 1 lb 75% lean ground beef
- 1 lb 72% lean ground pork
- ⅓ cup shredded Parmesan cheese
- 1 tsp granulated garlic
- 1 tsp granulated onion
- 1 tsp salt
- 1 tsp black pepper
- 8 oz mozzarella cheese, cut into small cubes
- 1 tbsp olive oil

Directions:
1. Preheat the oven to 350°F.
2. Combine beef, pork, Parmesan cheese, onion, garlic, salt, and pepper in a small bowl. Mix everything well until thoroughly combined.
3. Divide the beef mixture into 24 equal-sized portions and roughly shape it into balls with your hands (moisten your hands with water or olive oil to make things easier).
4. Now push a cube of mozzarella cheese into the center of each meatball and reshape to make sure that cheese is completely covered.
5. Use a large skillet to heat the olive oil over medium heat. Add meatballs to hot oil and brown on all sides. It is not necessary to wait until they are thoroughly cooked.
6. Arrange meatballs on a baking sheet in a single layer and bake for 30 minutes, turning the balls over once as they cook.
7. Remove from the oven and serve warm.
8. Enjoy!

Mediterranean Roll-Ups (Fat Bombs)

Time: 10 minutes
Serving Size: 2 fat bombs

Prep Time: 5 minutes

Cook Time: 5 minutes

Nutritional Facts/Info:

Calories 135

Carbs 1.8 g

Fat 12.6 g

Protein 3.5 g

Ingredients:
- 1 large egg
- 1 tbsp extra-virgin olive oil
- ⅛ tsp sea salt
- 6 large kalamata olives, pitted
- 2 tbsp sun-dried tomatoes in oil
- ⅛ tsp red chili flakes
- ⅛ tsp dried parsley

Directions:
1. Use a small bowl to combine egg, olive oil, and salt and whisk until foam forms.
2. Heat a small nonstick skillet over high heat and pour in egg mixture, spreading it evenly so that it forms a thin, even layer.
3. Once the first side is cooked, at about 1 minute, flip the frittata with the aid of a plate or a lid.
4. Cook until golden on the bottom, about 2 more minutes. Remove frittata to a plate.
5. Use a small food processor to mix olives, tomatoes, chili flakes, and parsley until well chopped and blended. This should take about 30 seconds.
6. Spread the olive paste on top of the frittata in an even layer.
7. Roll frittata into a tight roll, cut into 2 pieces and serve immediately.
8. Enjoy!

Buffalo Chicken Fingers

Time: 40 minutes
Serving Size: 4 servings

Prep Time: 10 minutes

Cook Time: 30 minutes

Nutritional Facts/Info:

Calories 839

Carbs 15.7 g

Fat 47.7 g

Protein 81 g

Ingredients:
- 2 cups almond flour
- 1 tsp salt
- 1 tsp black pepper
- 1 tsp dried parsley
- 2 large eggs
- 2 tbsps full-fat canned coconut milk
- 2 lbs chicken tenders
- 1½ cups Frank's RedHot Buffalo sauce

Directions:
1. Preheat the oven to 350°F.
2. Combine almond flour, salt, pepper, and parsley in a medium bowl and set aside.
3. Beat the eggs and coconut milk together in a separate medium bowl.
4. Dip each chicken tender into the egg mixture and then coat completely with almond flour mixture.
5. Place the coated chicken tenders spread out on the baking tray.
6. Bake for 30 minutes, flipping once during cooking. Let cool slightly.
7. Place chicken tenders in a large bowl and add buffalo sauce.
8. Toss to coat.
9. Serve, and enjoy!

Chorizo-Stuffed Jalapenos

Time: 35 minutes
Serving Size: 6 fat bombs

Prep Time: 10 minutes

Cook Time: 25 minutes

Nutritional Facts/Info:

Calories 219

Carbs 2.2 g

Fat 18.0 g

Protein 8.9 g

Ingredients:
- 1 tbsp olive oil
- ¼ medium yellow onion, peeled and minced
- 6 oz pork chorizo sausage
- 4 oz (½ cup) cream cheese, softened to room temperature
- 3 medium jalapeño peppers, seeded and sliced in half
- 3 slices no-sugar-added bacon, sliced in half horizontally

Directions:
1. Preheat the oven to 375°F.
2. Add olive oil to a medium skillet over medium heat and sweat onions for 2 minutes.
3. Add chorizo to the skillet and cook for another 3–5 minutes and drain the mixture.
4. Use a medium mixing bowl, whip cream cheese with a hand mixer until softened.
5. Fold in the sausage and onion mixture with a spatula.
6. Stuff each pepper half with cream cheese mixture.
7. Wrap 1 bacon slice around each stuffed pepper in a spiral motion, making sure that you cover the cream cheese mixture underneath.
8. Bake for 10–15 minutes or until bacon becomes crispy and cream cheese mixture underneath bubbles through and turns slightly brown.
9. Serve warm, and enjoy!

Onion Rings

Time: 30 minutes
Serving Size: 2 servings

Prep Time: 10 minutes

Cook Time: 20 minutes

Nutritional Facts/Info:

Calories 246

Carbs 53.6 g

Fat 12.6 g

Protein 16.8 g

Ingredients:
- 2 medium white onions, peeled and sliced into ½" rings
- 4 large eggs
- ⅓ cup full-fat canned coconut milk
- 1 cup pork rinds, crushed
- ¾ cup grated Parmesan cheese
- 1 cup coconut flour

Directions:
1. Preheat the oven to 425°F.
2. Break onion rings apart, removing smaller inside pieces and reserving only the rings.
3. Whisk together eggs and coconut milk in a medium bowl. Combine crushed pork rinds and Parmesan cheese in a separate medium bowl. Place coconut flour in a third medium bowl.
4. Dip each onion ring in coconut flour, then egg wash, then pork rind mixture. Repeat this process to double coat onion rings.
5. Line onion rings on a baking rack and bake for 15–20 minutes or until onion rings are golden and crispy.

Peanut Butter Power Granola

Time: 40 minutes
Serving Size: 12 servings

Prep Time: 10 minutes

Cook Time: 30 minutes

Nutritional Facts/Info:

Calories 338

Carbs 9.74 g

Fat 30.08 g

Protein 9.36 g

Ingredients:
- 1 ½ cups almonds
- 1 ½ cups pecans
- 1 cup shredded coconut or almond flour
- ¼ cup sunflower seeds
- ⅓ cup Swerve Sweetener
- ⅓ cup vanilla whey protein powder OR collagen protein powder
- ⅓ cup peanut butter
- ¼ cup butter
- ¼ cup water

Directions:
1. Preheat the oven to 300°F.
2. Tuck parchment paper into a large rimmed baking sheet.
3. Use a food processor to process almonds and pecans until they look like coarse crumbs with some larger pieces.
4. Now transfer them to a large bowl and stir in shredded coconut, sunflower seeds, vanilla protein powder, and sweetener.
5. Use a microwave-safe bowl to melt the peanut butter and butter together in the microwave.
6. Pour the melted peanut butter mixture into the nut mixture and toss it around before giving it a good stir.
7. Then stir in water and continue as the mixture clumps together.
8. Spread mixture evenly on the prepared baking sheet and bake for 30 minutes, stirring halfway through.
9. Remove and let cool completely.
10. Serve, and enjoy!

Keto Brownie Bark

Time: 45 minutes
Serving Size: 12 servings

Prep Time: 15 minutes

Cook Time: 30 minutes

Nutritional Facts/Info:

Calories 98

Carbs 4.3 g

Fat 8.3 g

Protein 2.4 g

Ingredients:
- 1/2 cup almond flour
- 1/2 tsp baking powder
- 1/4 tsp salt
- 2 large egg whites room temperature
- 1/2 cup Swerve sweetener granular
- 3 tbsp cocoa powder
- 1 tsp instant coffee (optional, intensifies chocolate flavors)
- 1/4 cup butter melted
- 1 tbsp heavy whipping cream
- 1/2 tsp vanilla
- 1/3 cups sugar-free chocolate chips

Directions:
1. Preheat the oven to 325°F.
2. Line a baking sheet with parchment paper and grease the parchment paper.
3. Use a small bowl to whisk together the almond flour, baking powder, and salt.
4. Use a large bowl to beat the egg whites until frothy, then pour in the sweetener, cocoa powder, and instant coffee until smooth, and then beat in melted butter, cream and vanilla.
5. Beat in the almond flour mixture until well combined.
6. Spread the batter onto the greased parchment into a rectangle about 12 by 8 inches. Sprinkle with the chocolate chips.
7. Bake for 18 minutes, until puffed and set.
8. Now remove the sheet from the oven, turn the oven off and let it cool for 15 minutes.
9. Use a sharp knife or pizza wheel to cut into 2-inch squares, but make sure that you don't separate.
10. Return to the warm oven for 5 to 10 minutes to crisp up slightly.
11. Remove, let cool completely and then break into squares.
12. Serve, and enjoy!

Coconut Chocolate Chip Cookies – Low Carb and Gluten-Free

Time: 30 minutes
Serving Size:

Prep Time: 15 minutes

Cook Time: 15 minutes

Nutritional Facts/Info:

Calories 238

Carbs 8.18 g

Fat 21.59 g

Protein 4.39 g

Ingredients:
- 1 1/4 cups almond flour
- 3/4 cups finely shredded unsweetened coconut
- 1 tsp baking powder
- 1/2 tsp salt
- 1/2 cup butter softened
- 1/2 cup Swerve Sweetener you can use another erythritol, but I can't guarantee the same results
- 2 tsp Yacon syrup or molasses optional
- 1/2 tsp vanilla extract
- 1 large egg

- 1/3 cup sugar-free chocolate chips or Homemade Sugar-Free Chocolate

Directions:
1. Preheat the oven to 325°F.
2. Dress a large baking sheet in parchment paper or a silicone mat.
3. Use a medium bowl to whisk together almond flour, coconut, baking powder, and salt.
4. Use a large bowl to cream butter with Swerve Sweetener and molasses.
5. Then beat in the vanilla and egg until well combined.
6. Beat in flour mixture until dough is well mixed.
7. Now add and stir in the sugar-free chocolate chips or homemade sugar-free chocolate chips.
8. Shape dough into a 1 1/2-inch ball and place 2 inches apart on the prepared baking sheet.
9. Press each ball with the heel of your hand to 1/4 inch thickness.
10. Bake for 12 to 15 minutes, until just beginning to brown and barely firm to the touch.
11. Remove from the oven and let cool completely on the pan.
12. Serve, and enjoy!

Classic Blueberry Scones

Time: 40 mins
Serving Size: 12 servings

Prep Time: 15 minutes

Cook Time: 25 minutes

Nutritional Facts/Info:

Calories 153

Carbs 7.21 g

Fat 12.15 g

Protein 5.55 g

Ingredients:
- 2 cups almond flour
- 1/3 cup Swerve Sweetener
- 1/4 cup coconut flour
- 1 tbsp baking powder
- 1/4 tsp salt
- 2 large eggs
- 1/4 cup heavy whipping cream
- 1/2 tsp vanilla extract
- 3/4 cup fresh blueberries

Directions:
1. Preheat the oven to 325°F.
2. Line a large baking sheet with parchment or a silicone mat.
3. Use a large bowl to throw together the almond flour, sweetener, coconut flour, baking powder, and salt.
4. Stir in the eggs, whipping cream, and vanilla, and mix until the dough begins to come together.
5. Now add the blueberries and carefully work them into the dough.
6. Put the dough together and place it onto the prepared baking sheet.
7. Pat into a rough rectangle about 10 by 8 inches.
8. Use a sharp large knife to cut into 6 squares.
9. Then cut each of those squares diagonally into two triangles. Gently lift the scones and distribute them around the pan.
10. Bake for 20 to 25 minutes, until it feels firm to the touch and turns golden. Remove and let cool.
11. Serve, and enjoy!

Classic Chocolate Cake Donuts

Time: 33 minutes
Serving Size: 8 donuts

Prep Time: 15 minutes

Cook Time: 18 minutes

Nutritional Facts/Info:

Calories 123

Carbs 4.68 g

Fat 9.2 g

Protein 4.43 g

Ingredients:
Donuts
- 1/3 cup coconut flour
- 1/3 cup Swerve Sweetener
- 3 tbsp cocoa powder
- 1 tsp baking powder
- 1/4 tsp salt
- 4 large eggs
- 1/4 cup butter melted
- 1/2 tsp vanilla extract
- 6 tbsp brewed coffee or water coffee intensifies the chocolate flavor

Glaze:

- 1/4 cup powdered Swerve sweetener
- 1 tbsp cocoa powder
- 1 tbsp heavy cream
- 1/4 tsp vanilla extract
- 1 1/2 to 2 tbsp water

Directions:
Donuts:
1. Preheat the oven to 325°F.
2. Then grease a donut pan very well.
3. Use a medium bowl to whisk together the sweetener, cocoa powder, coconut flour, baking powder, and salt.
4. Now stir in the eggs, the melted butter, and the vanilla extract, then stir in the fragrant cold coffee or the decaffeinated option of water until well combined.
5. Pour the batter into the wells of the donut pan. Create a steady stream of batches if your pans are too small for all the batter.
6. Let the batter harden away for 16 to 20 minutes, allowing it to reach a point where they are firm and springy to the touch.
7. Take care when removing them from the oven, and practice self-control by letting them cool for 10 minutes. Turn them onto a cooling rack to let them reach munching temperature.

Glaze:
8. Use a medium shallow bowl to whisk together the powdered sweetener and cocoa powder, adding in the vanilla and cream to complete the whisking.
9. Add just enough water to create a thin "dippable" consistency, but careful not to make it too watery.
10. Dip the top of each donut into the glaze and let set, for about 30 minutes.
11. Serve, and enjoy!

Homemade Caramel Frappuccino

Time: 5 minutes
Serving Size: 1 large frappuccino or 2 small frappuccinos

Prep Time: 5 minutes

Nutritional Facts/Info:

Calories 273

Carbs 2.99 g

Fat 27.4 g

Protein 2.15 g

Ingredients:
- 1 1/2 cups crushed ice
- 1/2 cup unsweetened almond milk
- 1/4 cup heavy whipping cream
- 1 packet Starbucks VIA© Ready Brew Coffee or 1 tsp instant espresso powder
- 2 tbsp powdered Swerve Sweetener
- 1/4 tsp caramel extract
- Lightly sweetened whipped cream for topping

Directions:
1. Use a high-powered blender to combine ice, almond milk, whipping cream, coffee, stevia extract, and caramel flavor.
2. Blend everything until smooth and top with whipped cream.
3. Serve, and enjoy!

Homemade Graham Crackers

Time: 1 hr 5 minutes
Serving Size: 10 servings

Prep Time: 15 minutes

Cook Time: 50 minutes

Nutritional Facts/Info:

Calories 156

Carbs 6.21 g

Fat 13.35 g

Protein 5.21 g

Ingredients:
- 2 cups almond flour
- 1/3 cup Swerve Brown (or 1/3 cup regular Swerve and 2 tsp molasses or Yacon syrup)
- 2 tsp cinnamon
- 1 tsp baking powder
- pinch salt
- 1 large egg
- 2 tbsp butter melted
- 1 tsp vanilla extract

Directions:
1. For the crackers: Preheat the oven to 300°F.
2. Use a large bowl to whisk together almond flour, sweetener, cinnamon, baking powder, and salt.
3. Add in the egg, melted butter, molasses, and vanilla extract until dough comes together.
4. Turn dough out onto a large piece of parchment paper or a silicone liner and pat it into a rough rectangle.
5. Top with another piece of parchment.
6. Roll out the dough as evenly as possible to about 1/8 to 1/4-inch thickness.
7. Remove the top parchment and use a sharp knife or a pizza wheel to score into squares of about 2" x 2" inches.
8. Then transfer the entire piece of parchment onto a baking sheet.
9. Bake for 20 to 30 minutes, until just beginning to brown and firm up.
10. Remove crackers and let cool for 30 minutes, then break up along score marks. Return to the warm oven (with the oven off . . . if it's cooled down too much, turn it on and set the temperature at no higher than 200°F).
11. Let them sit for another 30 minutes or so, then cool completely (they will crisp up as they cool).
12. Serve, and enjoy!

Keto Cinnamon Roll Biscotti

Time: 1 hour 20 minutes
Serving Size: 12 biscotti

Prep Time: 20 minutes

Cook Time: 1 hour

Nutritional Facts/Info:

Calories 133

Carbs 4 g

Fat 12 g

Protein 4 g

Ingredients:
Filling/Topping:
- 2 tbsp Swerve Sweetener
- 1 tsp ground cinnamon

Biscotti:
- 2 cups almond flour Honeyville
- 1/3 cup Swerve Sweetener
- 1 tsp baking powder
- 1/2 tsp xanthan gum
- 1/4 tsp salt
- 1/4 cup melted butter plus 1 tbsp for brushing biscotti
- 1 large egg

- 1 tsp vanilla extract

Glaze:
- 1/4 cup powdered Swerve Sweetener
- 2 tbsp heavy cream
- 1/2 tsp vanilla
- Instructions

Directions:
1. For the filling: combine sweetener and cinnamon in a small bowl and set aside.
2. Preheat the oven to 325°F.
3. Line a baking sheet with parchment paper.
4. Use a large bowl to whisk together almond flour, sweetener, baking powder, xanthan gum, and salt.
5. Then stir in 1/4 cup butter, egg, and vanilla extract until dough forms well.
6. Turn dough onto a prepared baking sheet and divide it in half.
7. Now form each half into a rectangle about 10 by 4 inches. Making sure that both halves are similar in size and shape.
8. Sprinkle one half with about 2/3 of the cinnamon filling.
9. Top with the other half of the dough and seal the seams and smooth the top.
10. Bake for 25 minutes or until lightly browned and just firm to the touch.
11. Then remove from the oven and brush with remaining melted butter, then sprinkle with remaining cinnamon mixture.
12. Allow them to cool for 30 minutes and reduce oven temperature to 250F.

13. Then use a sharp knife to cut the log into about 15 slices (a straight up and down motion works better than sawing back and forth).
14. Place slices back on the baking sheet cut-side down and bake for 15 minutes, then flip over and bake for another 15 minutes. Turn off the oven and let sit inside until cool.
15. For the glaze: whisk powdered sweetener with cream and vanilla extract until smooth. Drizzle over cooled biscotti.
16. Serve, and enjoy!

Raspberry Lemonade Smoothies

Time: 5 minutes
Serving Size: 4 servings

Prep Time: 5 minutes

Nutritional Facts/Info:

Calories 284

Carbs 6.6 g

Fat 21.9 g

Protein 14.4 g

Ingredients:
- 1 cup coconut milk
- 3/4 cup frozen raspberries
- 1/2 cup heavy whipping cream (or more coconut milk for dairy-free)
- 1/3 cup freshly squeezed lemon juice
- 1/4 cup powdered Swerve Sweetener more if you like it sweeter or sweetener of choice
- 1/4 cup collagen peptides
- 1 tsp lemon zest
- 2 cups ice

Directions:
1. Use a blender to combine all the ingredients and blend until smooth.
2. Divide between 4 glasses.
3. Serve, and enjoy!

Keto Smoothie

Time: 5 minutes
Serving Size: 4 servings

Prep Time: 5 minutes

Nutritional Facts/Info:

Calories 426

Carbs 41.3 g

Fat 30.1 g

Protein 4.4 g

Ingredients:
- 1 1/2 cups frozen strawberries
- 1 1/2 cups frozen raspberries, plus more for garnish (optional)
- 1 cup frozen blackberries
- 2 cup coconut milk
- 1 cup baby spinach
- unsweetened shaved coconut, for garnish (optional)

Directions:
1. Use a blender to combine all the ingredients (except for coconut) and blend until smooth.
2. Then divide between cups and top with raspberries and coconut.

Chocolate Keto Protein Shake

Time: 10 minutes
Serving Size: 1 serving

Prep Time: 10 minutes

Nutritional Facts/Info:

Calories 645 | Carbs 25.8 g | Fat 62.4 g | Protein 13 g

Ingredients:
- 3/4 cup almond milk
- 1/2 cup ice
- 2 tbsps almond butter
- 2 tbsps unsweetened cocoa powder
- 2 to 3 tbsps keto-friendly sugar substitute to taste (such as Swerve)
- 1 tbsp chia seeds, plus more for serving
- 2 tbsp hemp seeds, plus more for serving
- 1/2 tbsp pure vanilla extract
- pinch kosher salt

Directions:
1. Fill up a blender with all the ingredients, and get those blades spinning by blending it to a smooth consistency.
2. Then pour the shake into a glass and create that Instagram-worthy shot with more chia and hemp seeds.
3. Serve, and enjoy!

Chapter 7: 30-day Meal Prep for Beginners and 7-day Exercise Plan

Meal Plan

Week 1

Monday
Breakfast: Detox Tea
Lunch: Ham and Cheese Keto Stromboli
Dinner: Easy Chicken Cordon Bleu Casserole
Snack: Oven-baked Bacon Chips
Tuesday
Breakfast: Egg White Spinach Omelet
Lunch: Prosciutto, Caramelized Onion, & Parmesan Braid
Dinner: Low-Carb Keto Indian Butter Chicken
Snack: Grain-Free Amaretto Cookies
Wednesday
Breakfast: Bacon Frittata
Lunch: Spaghetti Squash with Meatballs
Dinner: Cheese Fathead Pizza Crust
Snack: Keto Guacamole
Thursday:
Breakfast: Cheese & Onion Quiche
Lunch: Easy Shrimp Avocado Salad with Tomatoes
Dinner: Beef Chili Recipe (Beanless Chili)
Snack: Keto Fudge Brownies
Friday
Breakfast: Cheese & Onion Quiche
Lunch: Baked Grill Chicken with Feta and Dill
Dinner: Easy Keto Bacon Cheeseburger Skillet.
Snack: Grain-Free Ameretto Cookies
Saturday
Breakfast: Keto French Toast
Lunch: Air Fryer Turkey Meatballs
Dinner: Keto Chicken in Lemon Cream Sauce
Snack: Low-Carb Cheese Crackers
Sunday
Breakfast: Crunchy Keto Cereal with Strawberries
Lunch: Cucumber Tomato Salad
Dinner: Keto Buffalo Chicken Quesadilla
Snack: Keto Sugar-Free Chocolate Pudding

Week 2

Monday
Breakfast: Homemade Sage Sausage Patties
Lunch: Cheddar Broccoli Soup
Dinner: Keto Bacon Cheeseburger Casserole
Snack: Keto Low Carb Lemon Blueberry Bread
Tuesday
Breakfast: Cinnamon Roll Cereal
Lunch: Avocado Tuna Melt Bites
Dinner: Italian Cheese Stuffed Meatloaf
Snack: Healthy Avocado Chocolate Cookies
Wednesday
Breakfast: Eggs Florentine Casserole
Lunch: Homemade Keto Caesar Salad
Dinner: Keto Jalapeno Popper Stuffed Chicken
Snack: Keto Fermented Dill Pickles
Thursday
Breakfast: Keto Breakfast Grits
Lunch: Grilled Tuna Salad with Garlic Dressing
Dinner: Keto Chicken Parmesan
Snack: Buffalo Cauliflower Bites
Friday
Breakfast: Keto Mushroom Omelet
Lunch: Keto Cloud Bread
Dinner: Keto Ham and Cheese Crustless Quiche
Snack: Keto Crackers
Saturday
Breakfast: Keto Lemon Chia Pudding
Lunch: Ketofied Chick-Fil-A Chicken
Dinner: Keto Garlic Dusted Dinner Rolls
Snack: Garlic Bacon Dip
Sunday
Breakfast: Keto Crepes
Lunch: Keto Roasted Pumpkin & Halloumi Salad
Dinner: Keto One Skillet Chicken in Lemon Cream Sauce
Snack: Chicken Skin Crisps with Spicy Avocado Cream (Fat Bombs)

Week 3

Monday
Breakfast: Keto Eggs Benedict
Lunch: Keto Meaty Mediterranean Lunch Bowls
Dinner: Keto Mexican Zucchini and Beef
Snack: Cheesy Meatballs
Tuesday
Breakfast: Keto Granola Cereal
Lunch: Keto Crispy Ginger Mackerel Lunch Bowl
Dinner: Hamburger Sausage and Broccoli Alfredo
Snack: Mediterranean Roll-Ups (Fat Bombs)
Wednesday
Breakfast: Keto Meal Replacement Shake
Lunch: Keto Bacon Cheeseburger Kebabs
Dinner: Keto Cauliflower Pizza Crust
Snack: Buffalo Chicken Fingers
Thursday
Breakfast: Huevos Rancheros
Lunch: Keto Tuna Cheese Melt
Dinner: Bacon Cheeseburger Soup
Snack: Chorizo-Stuffed Jalapenos
Friday
Breakfast: Keto Breakfast Enchiladas
Lunch: Keto Thai Fish Curry
Dinner: Lasagna Stuffed Portobellos
Snack: Onion Rings
Saturday
Breakfast: Keto Chicken and Waffle Sandwiches
Lunch: Creamy Keto Fish Casserole
Dinner: Pesto Spinach Artichoke Chicken Bake
Snack: Peanut Butter Power Granola
Sunday
Breakfast: Keto Pepperoni Pizza Quiche
Lunch: Keto Meat Pie
Dinner: Bacon Ranch Chicken Crust Pizza
Snack: Keto Brownie Bark

Week 4

Monday
Breakfast: Gooey Keto Cinnamon Rolls
Lunch: Keto Lasagna
Dinner: Moroccan Meatballs
Snack: Coconut Chocolate Chip Cookies—Low Carb and Gluten-Free
Tuesday
Breakfast: Keto Lemon Sugar Poppy Seed Scones
Lunch: Keto Asian Cabbage Stir-Fry
Dinner: Keto Tacos
Snack: Classic Blueberry Scones
Wednesday
Breakfast: Bacon Kale and Tomato Frittata
Lunch: Italian Keto Meatballs with Mozzarella Cheese
Dinner: Low Carb Big Mac Bites
Snack: Classic Chocolate Cake Donuts
Thursday
Breakfast: Vegan Keto Scramble
Lunch: Easy Low-Carb Cauliflower Mac 'n Cheese
Dinner: Keto Fried Chicken in the Air Fryer
Snack: Homemade Caramel Frappuccino
Friday
Breakfast: Keto Sausage Gravy and Biscuit Bake
Lunch: Cobb Salad
Dinner: Keto Easy Herb-Roasted Turkey
Snack: Homemade Graham Crackers
Saturday
Breakfast: No-tatoes Bubble and Squeak
Lunch: Keto Instant Pot Soup (Low Carb)
Dinner: Pork Fried Rice
Snack: Keto Cinnamon Roll Biscotti
Sunday
Breakfast: Lemon Raspberry Sweet Rolls
Lunch: Easy Keto Beef Tacos
Dinner: Roast Pork Belly
Snack: Raspberry Lemonade Smoothies

Exercise Plan

Although the keto diet is sufficient on its own to help you lose weight. It is helpful to keep an active lifestyle, to retain weight loss, and for your overall health. The following weekly exercise plan is just a guideline you can follow to help you get comfortable with exercising. The exercises are safe and do not apply too much pressure on the joints.

Monday
15 minutes' walk x 2
Taking a walk outside can help improve your strength, balance, and flexibility. You can opt to walk on a treadmill or take a walk at a park or in your neighborhood. This small effort is enough to get the heart pumping gently and your muscles loosened.

Tuesday
30 minutes cycling
This is a little more intense cardio workout. If you have a bicycle at home that has been sitting in the garage, how about you take it out for a spin? You do not have to go at a particular pace, just making the regular cycling movements will help strengthen your legs and the fresh pumping of blood will clear your head.

Wednesday
30 minutes swimming/water aerobics
If you struggle with joint pain, this will become a favorite for you. Water keeps the body floating, working against gravity. Therefore, you get to do a lot of physical movement without feeling the pull to the ground.

Thursday
Rest
If this is your first week, by Thursday you will feel the need to rest your muscles. As the weeks progress and your fitness

improve, it will be helpful to increase the intensity of your workouts.

Friday

30 minutes' walk

By Friday, your body will have rested. You need to keep up the endurance by adding intensity. So going for a thirty-minute walk will do you good. If you have a fitness watch, you can track your duration even if you are at the mall running errands.

Saturday

30 minutes cycling/swimming/water aerobics

Again, this is similar to Wednesday's routine. However, here the intensity has been increased.

Sunday

Rest

You can use Sunday to rest and plan for the rest of the week.

Additional Exercises

Abdominal Contractions

These are great to get your mid-section working. The process may seem easy, but with them, these little efforts will build up to give great results.
1. First, take a deep breath and tighten your abdominal muscles.
2. Hold for 3 breaths and then release the contraction.
3. Repeat 10 times.

Wall Pushups

These simple exercises are great for maintaining upper arm strength, as well as shoulder and chest strength. They are easy to do, all you need is a firm wall and some gripping shoes, then you are good to go.
1. Stand about 3 feet away from a wall, facing the wall, with your feet shoulder-width apart.
2. Lean forward and put your hands flat on the wall, parallel with your shoulders. Your body should be in plank position, with your spine straight, not sagging or arched.
3. Lower your body toward the wall and then push back.
4. Repeat 10 times.

Pelvic Tilts

Here is an exercise that helps with lower body stiffness. This exercise helps strengthen the upper leg area and the lower back. If you have a problem with lower back stiffness this is the exercise you need. It will relieve your muscle tension, giving you relief.

1. Take a deep breath, tighten your buttocks, and tilt your hips slightly forward.
2. Hold for about 3 seconds.
3. Now tilt your hips back, and hold for 3 seconds. (It's a very subtle movement.)
4. Repeat 8 to 12 times.

Reference

Allrecipes. (n.d.). *Keto Diet Recipes.* [online] Available at: https://www.allrecipes.com/recipes/22959/healthy-recipes/keto-diet/ [Accessed 7 Dec. 2020].

Diet Doctor. (n.d.). *500+ Easy Keto Recipes – Meals, Bread & More.* [online] Available at: https://www.dietdoctor.com/low-carb/keto/recipes.

Healthline. (2017). *10 Fantastic Keto Recipes.* [online] Available at: https://www.healthline.com/health/food-nutrition/keto-recipes.

Keto A to Z. (2020). *Home.* [online] Available at: https://ketoa2z.com/?fbclid=IwAR1r5r2EPumD3AT6uJSg6bvRacvJ2hST1g8LkaUnQUO-zWh7GUtDRRP2TCg [Accessed 7 Dec. 2020].

Printed in Great Britain
by Amazon